THIRD EDITION

Blood
Collection

A Short Course

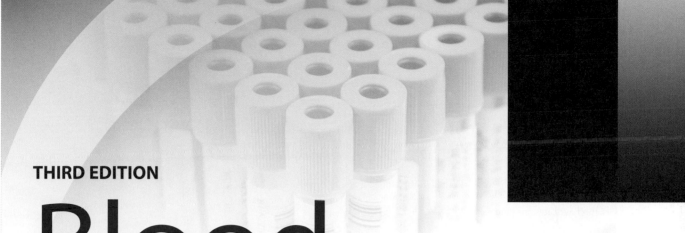

THIRD EDITION

Blood Collection

A Short Course

Marjorie Schaub Di Lorenzo, MT(ASCP)SH

Phlebotomy Technician Program Coordinator
Health Professions
Nebraska Methodist College – The Josie Harper Campus
Omaha, Nebraska

Susan King Strasinger, DA, MT(ASCP)

Faculty Associate
The University of West Florida
Pensacola, Florida

F.A. Davis Company • Philadelphia

F. A. Davis Company
1915 Arch Street
Philadelphia, PA 19103
www.fadavis.com

Printed in the United States of America

Last digit indicates print number: 10 9 8 7 6 5 4 3 2 1

Senior Acquisitions Editor: Christa Fratantoro
Director of Content Development: George W. Lang
Developmental Editor: Karen Carter
Design and Illustration Manager: Carolyn O'Brien

As new scientific information becomes available through basic and clinical research, recommended treatments and drug therapies undergo changes. The author(s) and publisher have done everything possible to make this book accurate, up to date, and in accord with accepted standards at the time of publication. The author(s), editors, and publisher are not responsible for errors or omissions or for consequences from application of the book, and make no warranty, expressed or implied, in regard to the contents of the book. Any practice described in this book should be applied by the reader in accordance with professional standards of care used in regard to the unique circumstances that may apply in each situation. The reader is advised always to check product information (package inserts) for changes and new information regarding dose and contraindications before administering any drug. Caution is especially urged when using new or infrequently ordered drugs.

Library of Congress Cataloging-in-Publication Data

Names: Di Lorenzo, Marjorie Schaub, 1953- , author. | Strasinger, Susan King, author.
Title: Blood collection : a short course / Marjorie Schaub Di Lorenzo, Susan King Strasinger.
Description: Third edition. | Philadelphia : F.A. Davis Company, [2016] | Preceded by Blood collection / Marjorie Schaub Di Lorenzo, Susan King Strasinger. 2nd ed. c2010. | Includes bibliographical references and index.
Identifiers: LCCN 2016000518 | ISBN 9780803646070
Subjects: | MESH: Phlebotomy—methods | Phlebotomy—instrumentation | Blood Specimen Collection—methods | Blood Specimen Collection—instrumentation
Classification: LCC RB45.15 | NLM QY 25 | DDC 616.07/561—dc23 LC record available at http://lccn.loc.gov/2016000518

To my parents, Arthur and Charlotte Schaub

MSD

To Harry, you will always be my Editor-in-Chief

SKS

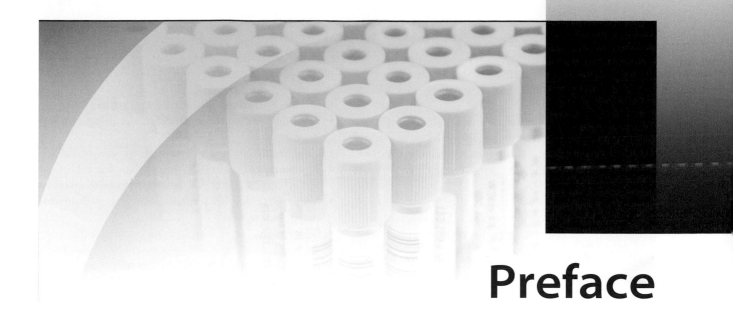

Preface

This revised short course textbook is designed to provide practicing health-care personnel with concise current information on the correct and safe techniques and equipment to collect quality blood samples with minimal patient discomfort. The purpose of the book, *Blood Collection: A Short Course*, Edition 3, is primarily for the cross-training and continuing education of health-care professionals currently performing blood collection or those who anticipate performing blood and other specimen collections in the future. Today's concept of developing health-care teams to help streamline patient care has evolved to encompass the cross-training of nurses, respiratory therapists, radiographers, medical assistants, certified nursing assistants, medical laboratory scientists and technicians, and others. Blood collection has become a major part of this cross-training.

In an attempt to anticipate the needs of the various health professions, this textbook has enhanced many topics to include:

- Quality management
- Regulatory agencies, such as CLIA, CAP, TJC, and COLA
- Safety and infection control
- HIPAA and legal considerations
- Hemostasis
- Collection techniques for capillary, venous, and arterial blood
- Vein selection and alternate sites
- Vascular access devices
- Newborn screening

- Types of blood required for specific lab tests
- Purpose of laboratory tests and body system correlation
- Types of collection tubes and the purpose of tube additives
- Order of draw
- Test-specific handling
- Complications and remedies
- Sample handling, storage, and transportation conditions
- Point of care testing
- Internet resources
- Review questions
- For Further Study questions for critical thinking stimulation
- Case Studies for practical application
- Full-color illustrations

In addition, *Blood Collection*, Edition 3, includes updated information on point-of-care testing, preexamination variables and the effect on the integrity of the sample, current ADA guidelines for the diagnosis of diabetes mellitus, arterial blood collection, and newborn bilirubin and newborn screening procedures. A new comprehensive appendix includes lab tests with the correct collection tube, special instructions, department for testing, and the clinical correlation. Covered also in the appendices are lab tests to correlate with the various body systems, the answers to the review questions, for further study questions, and case studies. Appendix D lists common abbreviations used in connection with the laboratory and blood collection. Information common to all health-care curriculums, such as safety precautions, anatomy and physiology, quality management, and patient-caregiver interactions, is covered only in the context of their relationship to the collection of blood samples.

This current comprehensive text provides a cost-effective, compact learning tool for phlebotomy short courses and is a perfect choice for continuing education programs and for health-care programs such as medical assisting, nursing, radiography, and medical laboratory science where blood collection may be integrated into the curriculum or job description. Coverage of the following topics is included in this edition:

- Blood collection equipment, including the newest safety devices
- Technical procedures for venipuncture, dermal puncture, and arterial puncture
- Special collection procedures, including access to central venous catheters and IV insertion and care, blood cultures, therapeutic drug monitoring, glucose tolerance tests, and point of care tests, neonatal bilirubin, newborn screening
- Sample handling, storage, and transport procedures
- Preexamination, examination, and postexamination variables
- Patient complications
- Technical complications
- Methods to ensure the quality of blood sample
- Correlation of laboratory tests and clinical disorders
- Quality management procedures required by laboratory regulatory agencies as they relate to phlebotomy

Note that all procedures are written to comply with the standards set forth by the Occupational Safety and Health Administration, The Joint Commission, and the Clinical and Laboratory Standards Institute.

Key features of the third edition include:

- **Learning objectives** to identify the important concepts of each chapter.
- **Key terms,** defined at the beginning of each chapter and bolded throughout the chapter.
- **Technical tips,** to avoid complications, such as hemoconcentration, nerve damage, hematomas and hemolysis.

- **Safety Tips** stressing extra safety precautions.
- **Procedure Boxes** to concisely illustrate and explain each step of all the procedures.
- **Review Questions** to test your knowledge.
- **For Further Study Questions** to develop critical-thinking skills.
- **Case Studies** to incorporate problem solving skills.
- **Performance evaluation checklists** for technical procedures to check your knowledge of each step.
- **Numerous color illustrations, photographs, diagrams, charts, and tables**
- **Bibiography** at the end of each chapter for your reference.
- **Internet Resources** for additional help.
- **Appendices** that include valuable reference information.

This text provides a quick reference with the most current updates for blood collection skills. Appendices list reference material, such as frequently ordered laboratory tests with the required types of anticoagulants and volume of blood required, special instructions, and the department where the test is performed. A summary of laboratory tests, their functions, and their clinical correlation is included. Answer keys for the review questions, for further study questions, and case studies also are available. A complete color tube guide for both the BD and the Vacuette systems list all the different types of collection tubes, the additives, number of inversions required, and laboratory uses of the tubes.

Available also to the users of the textbook is access to the Davis*Plus* website with interactive learning activities for both students and instructors. Students will have access to animations and videos on techniques for venipuncture and dermal puncture. Instructor's resources include a PowerPoint presentation for each chapter, lecture outline, competency checklists, discussion questions, and a complete test bank. We specifically designed this text to meet the needs of nurses and other health-care professionals who want and need to add a new blood collection competency or to reinforce past learned skills. It can be used to promote learning in academic settings, hospital-training sessions, or continuing education courses.

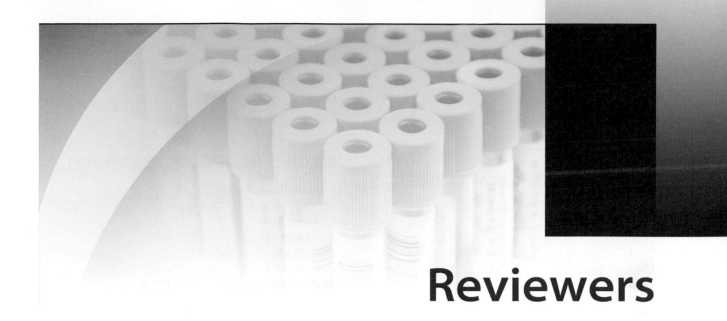

Reviewers

Rhonda Anderson, PBT(ASCP)CM

Program Manager/Instructor
CEHP Program
Environmental Health and Safety Department
Greenville Technical College
Greenville, South Carolina

Cynthia L. Banna, M.Ed., CLS, MLT(ASCP)HCM

Assistant Professor
Department of Allied Health
Community College of Rhode Island
Lincoln, Rhode Island

Pamela Christianson, CMA, Licensed and Certified Pharmacy Technician, BS

Program Director/Faculty
Department of Health Science
Great Falls College MSU
Great Falls , Montana

Vera Dauffenbach, EdD, MSN, RN

Associate Professor
Department of Nursing
Bellin College
Green Bay, Wisconsin

Penny Ewing, BS, CMA (AAMA)

Medical Assisting/Phlebotomy Instructor
Department of Medical Assisting/Phlebotomy
Gaston College
Dallas, North Carolina

Kristine Hayes, MAT, MLS(ASCP)CM

MLT & Phlebotomy program coordinator and
    Assistant professor
Department of Allied Health
Moberly Area Community College
Mexico, Missouri

Starra R. Herring, BSAH, BSHA, CMA(AAMA)-MA, AHI

Medical Assisting Program Director
Stanly Community College
Abelmarle, North Carolina

Patty Janousek, BSN, CRNI

IV Team
Methodist Hospital
Omaha, Nebraska

Rose Knapp, DNP, RN, APN-BC

Assistant Graduate Faculty/ Nurse Practitioner
  Program Coordinator
Department of Department of Nursing
Monmouth University
West Long Branch, New Jersey

Kristin Kuhlmann, PhD, APRN, FNP-BC

Assistant Professor, Director of WTAMU Health
  Partners Clinic
Department of Nursing
West Texas A & M University
Canyon, Texas

Jessica Lasiter, MHIM, MLS(ASCP)CM

Assistant Professor and Clinical Coordinator
Department of Medical Laboratory Science
University of Louisiana Monroe
Monroe, Louisiana

Diana Lee-Greene, RMA(AMT), MT, MBA

Program Coordinator
Department of Nursing and Health Occupations
Columbia Gorge Community College
The Dalles, Oregon

Jody Lynn Lester, MA

Chair
Department of Respiratory Care
Boise State University
Boise, Idaho

Barbara L. Marchelletta, RHIT, CMA, CPT, CPC

Program Director
Allied Health Department
MA Program
Beal College
Bangor, Maine

Claudine Matthews, RRT

Program Director
Department of Respiratory Therapy
Southern University at Shreveport
Shreveport, Louisiana

Linda J. McCown, PhD, MT(ASCP)

Chair and Associate Professor
Clinical Laboratory Science
University of Illinois Springfield
Springfield, Illinois

Pamela D. Meadows, MS, BSMT (ASCP)

Title Assistant Professor
Department of Clinical Laboratory Sciences
  Department
Marshall University
Huntington, West Virginia

Maile Nelson, BA, CMA, MLA

Clinical Coordinator/Faculty for Medical Laboratory
  and Medical Assisting Programs
Department of Allied Health Department
South Piedmont Community College
Monroe, North Carolina

Patricia A. Nolan, M.Ed., RRT

Assistant Professor
School of Health Professions
Community College of Baltimore County (CCBC)
Baltimore, Maryland

Jill Ogg-Gress, DNP MSN ARNP

Family Nurse Practitioner
Council Bluffs, Iowa

Susan Porterfield, PhD, FNP-c

Assistant Dean of Graduate Programs
Department of Nursing
Florida State University
Tallahassee, Florida

Maria Carina Quiogue Relopsa, RN

Nursing Educator
LPN Program
Preferred College of Nursing
Los Angeles, California

Catherine Marie Moran Robinson, MLT (CSMLS), MT (ASCP), MSc., MEd

Coordinator/Instructor Medical Laboratory Assistant and Medical Laboratory Technology Programs
Department of Allied Health
New Brunswick Community College
Saint John, New Brunswick
Canada

Georgette Rosenfeld, RRT, RN, PhD.

Department Chair
Department of Respiratory Care
Indian River State College
Fort Pierce, Florida

C. Thomas Somma, EdD

Associate Professor
Department of Medical Diagnostics and Translational Sciences
Old Dominion University
Norfolk, Virginia

Eric Staples, RN, DNP

Nursing Practice Consultant
Ancaster, Ontario
Canada

Lynne L. Steele, MS, MT(ASCP)Program Chair

Department of Medical Laboratory Technology
Oakton Community College
Des Plaines, Illinois

Debbie Sutherland, Certified Phlebotomist

Phlebotomy Program
Science Hill Tech Center
Johnson City, Tennessee

William D Wood, MAEd, RRT-NPS, RCP

Dean, Health Sciences
Department of Health Sciences
Wilkes Community College
Wilkesboro, North Carolina

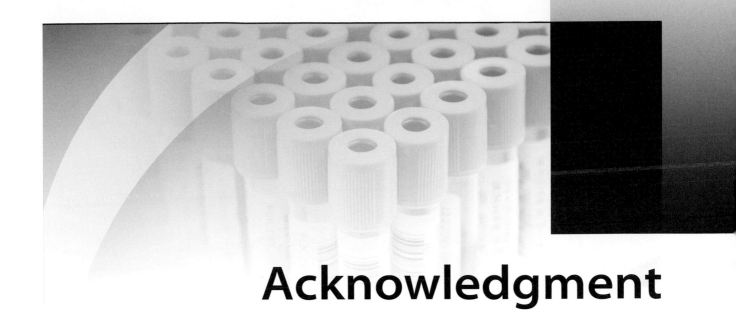

Acknowledgment

Many individuals gave of their time and expertise to make this third edition of *Blood Collection: A Short Course* and the accompanying ancillary activities possible. We wish to thank Patty Janousek, BSN,CRNI, IV Team, and the administration and staff at Methodist Hospital for their continued support. We are deeply grateful for the dedication of the staff at F.A. Davis, especially those with whom we have worked most closely: Karen Carter, Developmental Editor, George Lang, Director of Content Development, Elizabeth Stepchin, Project Editor, Elizabeth Bales, Developmental Editor of Electronic Products, and Christa Fratantoro, Senior Acquisitions Editor.

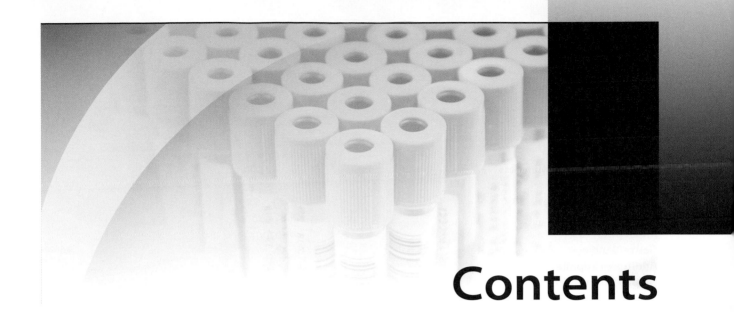

Contents

Appendix A

Appendix B

Appendix C

Appendix D

1

Introduction to Blood Collection

LEARNING OBJECTIVES

Upon completion of this chapter, the reader will be able to:

1.1 Recognize the importance of correct blood collection techniques in managing total patient care.

1.2 List the factors that influence the integrity of a blood sample.

1.3 State the purpose of regulations and legal considerations in blood collection.

1.4 Discuss safety precautions and infection control as related to blood collection.

1.5 Describe quality management in blood collection.

KEY TERMS

Aliquot A portion of a sample

Chain of Custody Documentation of the collection and handling of forensic samples

Clinical Laboratory Improvement Amendments (CLIA) Federal regulations governing laboratories that test human samples

Clinical and Laboratory Standards Institute (CLSI) Nonprofit organization that publishes standards and guidelines for clinical laboratory procedures

Healthcare–associated infection Infection acquired by a patient as the result of a hospital stay or an outpatient procedure

Health Insurance Portability and Accountability Act (HIPAA) Legislation that guarantees the privacy of individual health information

Preexamination Phase Processes that occur before testing of a specimen

Sample One or more parts taken from a system

Specimen Portion of a body fluid or tissue taken for examination such as an aliquot of plasma or serum

INTRODUCTION

The redesigning of the health-care system to obtain more efficient and cost-effective patient care has resulted in many changes in personnel responsibilities. One of the major changes has been the shifting of blood **sample** collection from phlebotomists based in the clinical laboratory to nurses and other health professionals that include certified nursing assistants, medical assistants, patient care technicians, respiratory therapists, radiographers, physician assistants, paramedics, and emergency medical technicians.

Consequently, many health-care personnel are now required to become proficient in a skill for which they have had little or no previous exposure. Like any other skill, collection of quality blood samples begins by obtaining the didactic knowledge associated with the procedure, and then continues with performing the procedure with assistance and supervision. All procedures are written in accordance with the current standards of the **Clinical and Laboratory Standards**

Institute (CLSI) and the current Occupational Safety & Health Administration (OSHA) guidelines and the Centers for Disease Control and Prevention (CDC) recommendations. Adhering to proper technique and continued practice then becomes the key to acquiring proficiency. Regular competency assessments are required to evaluate the blood collector's initial training and to ensure that the blood collector's performance continues to comply with the current standards.

IMPORTANCE OF CORRECT SAMPLE COLLECTION AND HANDLING

Laboratory testing of blood **specimens** is vital to the correct diagnosis, treatment, and monitoring of a patient's condition. Laboratory results constitute approximately 70 percent of the objective information used by health-care providers to diagnose and manage patient care and resolve patient health problems. The quality of a test result is only as good as the quality of the specimen analyzed. Test results from a suboptimal specimen can cause inappropriate treatment that can be potentially harmful to the patient, with death being the worst patient outcome. Conversely, reporting a test result as normal when in fact it was abnormal can cause the health-care provider to miss an abnormal patient condition and the necessity for reflective tests.

Although the primary concern of personnel collecting blood samples is understandably to obtain the sample, failure to adhere to the collection procedure can compromise the integrity of a successfully collected sample. Approximately 56 percent of laboratory error occurs during the **preexamination phase** of laboratory testing. Influencing factors are the responsibilities of the blood collector and include the following:

- Monitoring of sample ordering
- Correct patient identification
- Patient communication and safety
- Patient preparation
- Timing of collections
- Phlebotomy equipment
- Collection techniques
- Sample labeling
- Sample transportation to the laboratory
- Sample processing

These ancillary factors most frequently affect sample integrity, resulting in sample rejection by the laboratory. Therefore, emphasis in this course is placed on both technical and nontechnical factors that must be included in quality blood sample collection.

REGULATORY ISSUES

Health-care regulation systems include both governmental and public agencies. All agencies have the same goal, which is to provide safe and effective health care. The following agencies provide standards to ensure quality blood collection and laboratory testing procedures.

Clinical Laboratory Improvement Amendments

Laboratories are charged with the responsibility for reliable and timely test results by the **Clinical Laboratory Improvement Amendments (CLIA).** These are federal regulations administered by the Centers for Medicare & Medicaid Services (CMS) and the Food and Drug Administration (FDA) to stipulate that all laboratories that perform testing on human specimens for the purposes of diagnosis, prevention, treatment, monitoring, or screening must be licensed and obtain a certificate from the CMS. The FDA classifies laboratory tests as waived or nonwaived tests with regard to the skill level for personnel performing the tests. Tests are continually being developed and added to the waived test category. For an up-to-date listing of waived tests, refer to the CLIA website. Nonwaived testing is separated into the categories of moderate and high complexity. Provider-performed microscopy procedures (PPMP) must meet the moderate complexity requirements for proficiency testing, patient test management, quality control (QC), and quality assurance (QA) as required by the accreditation agency. **(See Box 1-1.)** Laboratories are subject to inspection every 2 years by CMS personnel or an accrediting agency recognized by CMS, including the College of American Pathologists (CAP), The Joint Commission (TJC), and the Commission on Laboratory Assessment (COLA). **(See Box 1-2.)**

Clinical and Laboratory Standards Institute (CLSI)

All laboratory procedures are written in accordance with the current standards of the **Clinical and Laboratory Standards Institute (CLSI).** The CLSI is an organization of representatives from the laboratory profession, industry, and government that develop and publish guidelines and standards for all areas of the laboratory, including blood collection. The responsibility of the CLSI is to ensure that all procedures are consistent with the current research and industry regulations.

BOX 1-1 CLIA Classifications

WAIVED TESTING

Tests considered easy to perform by following the manufacturer's instructions and that have little risk of error. No special training or education is required.

Example: Urine pregnancy test

PROVIDER-PERFORMED MICROSCOPY PROCEDURES (PPMP)

Microscopy tests performed by a physician, midlevel practitioner, or dentist.

Example: Microscopic urinalysis

MODERATE COMPLEXITY TESTS

Tests that require documentation of training in test principles, instrument calibration, periodic proficiency testing and competency assessment, and on-site inspections. Personnel performing moderate complexity tests must have a high school diploma.

Example: Automated complete blood count (CBC)

HIGH COMPLEXITY TESTS

Tests that require sophisticated instrumentation and a high degree of interpretation. Proficiency testing and on-site inspections are required. Personnel performing high complexity tests must have a formal education with a degree in clinical laboratory science.

Example: Urine culture and sensitivity

In accordance with these standards, guidelines for sample collection are published by the laboratory and should be available in all areas in which patient samples are collected. Personnel collecting samples should become familiar with these guidelines and refer to them or call the laboratory whenever they are unsure of a procedure. In a legal situation, they are considered the standards of care that should have been met.

LEGAL CONSIDERATIONS

Medical law regulates the conduct of members of the health-care professions. Understanding the activities

---

BOX 1-2 Accrediting Agencies

THE JOINT COMMISSION (TJC)

Independent, not-for-profit organization that accredits and certifies health-care organizations

COLLEGE OF AMERICAN PATHOLOGISTS (CAP)

Organization of board-certified pathologists that provide laboratory accreditation and proficiency testing for hospital laboratories

COMMISSION ON LABORATORY ASSESSMENT (COLA)

Physician-directed accrediting agency popular with physicians' office laboratories and independent laboratories

---

that can result in legal action can help to prevent them. The most common phlebotomy events that may initiate litigation include the following:

- Nerve injury
- Hemorrhage from an accidental arterial puncture or inadequate pressure to the vein
- Drawing from inappropriate locations (e.g., from the same side of the body that a mastectomy was done)
- Injuries occurring when a patient faints
- Wrong diagnosis or mistreatment of a patient because of sample collection errors
- Death of a patient caused by misidentification of a patient or sample

 TECHNICAL TIP 1-1

To avoid becoming involved in malpractice litigation, the blood collector must follow, at all times, the procedures that are written according to CLSI standards.

The Health Insurance Portability and Accountability Act (HIPAA)

The **Health Insurance Portability and Accountability Act (HIPAA)** of 1996 was created to protect the privacy of patients' health information. This legislation requires that the release of patient information must be kept to

the minimum required for care and that written patient consent to release the information must be obtained. All information acquired through the care of a patient must be kept confidential and given only to health professionals who have a medical need to know. Laboratory results may be given only to the health-care provider, and the patient must give permission to release the test results. HIPAA has mandated that health-care professionals become familiar with the information security standards and sign an agreement that indicates knowledge of the policies to control access and release of patient-identifiable health information. HIPAA violations that could involve litigation include the following:

- Accessing a patient's chart without a need to know
- Leaving results visible on a computer screen or printer
- Not logging off the computer, leaving it open for others to view patient results
- Giving patient results to a family member or other interested persons without the patient's consent

Patient Consent

The blood collector must explain the procedure that will be used to collect the blood sample, stressing that the patient's health-care provider ordered the test. The patient expects that the blood collector is competent in blood collection procedures and gives informed consent verbally or by extending the arm or rolling up the sleeve. Blood collectors may be legally liable for failing to offer information to patients and for not obtaining informed consent.

 TECHNICAL TIP 1-2

A patient has the right to refuse medical treatment, and this decision should be documented in the medical record.

Chain of Custody

When collecting a sample used for test results that may be used as evidence in legal proceedings, blood collectors must follow stated policies for collecting and handling the sample exactly according to policy. Documentation of sample handling, called the **chain of custody,** is essential. It begins with patient identification and continues until testing is completed and results are reported. Special forms are provided for the documentation. For each person handling the sample, documentation must include the date, the time, and the identification of the handler. Tests most frequently requested are blood alcohol and drug levels and DNA analysis.

SAFETY PRECAUTIONS AND INFECTION CONTROL

All personnel working or preparing to work in health care must be thoroughly knowledgeable about the many precautions necessary to protect both patients and providers. **Healthcare–associated infection (HAI)** refers to an infection acquired by a patient as the result of a health-care procedure. Infection control programs developed by the CDC have been developed to control HAIs. **Figure 1-1** provides an overall picture of the causes and procedures to prevent transmission of infection. Notice that each area can be related to blood collection.

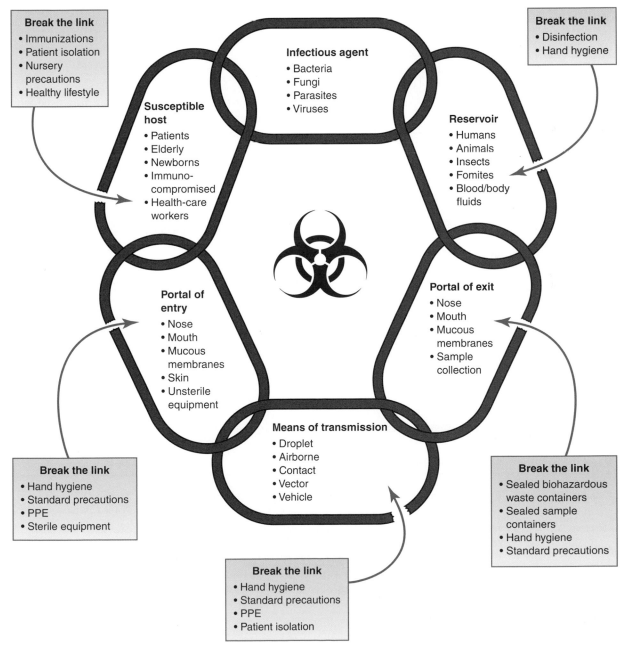

FIGURE 1-1 Chain of infection and safety practices related to the biohazard symbol. *(Reproduced with permission from Strasinger, S.K., and Di Lorenzo, M.S.: The Phlebotomy Textbook, ed. 3. Philadelphia, F.A. Davis, 2011.)*

In addition to the safety precautions specifically associated with blood collection, which are covered in this text, personnel must observe all standard precautions required in patient care. These include the following:

- Wearing appropriate personal protective equipment (PPE)
- Observation of isolation practices (**Table 1-1**)
- Hand sanitizing
- Using only needles with safety devices in the intended manner (Chapter 2)
- Disposal in a biohazard container of entire assembled tube holder and needle after use
- Recording all accidental needlesticks and exposures as required by the OSHA-mandated written exposure control plan. Postexposure prophylaxis (PEP) should be started when necessary.

 SAFETY TIP 1-1

Needles used for blood collection have a greater potential for transmitting bloodborne pathogens than do needles used for other purposes. Never hesitate to report *all* needlesticks.

- Disposal of contaminated materials in designated biohazard containers
- Decontamination of surfaces using an approved disinfectant, such as sodium hypochlorite (diluted 1:10, or 1:100 for routine decontamination) prepared daily and stored in a plastic bottle

- Observing transmission guidelines for blood collectors (**Box 1-3**)

Blood collection poses a serious risk for exposure to bloodborne pathogens, such as HIV, hepatitis B (HBV), and hepatitis C (HCV). HBV and HCV have been found to be stable in dried blood and blood products for approximately 7 days. Standard precautions must be strictly observed (**Fig. 1-2**). Workstation countertops, equipment, and telephones must be disinfected daily or when visually contaminated. PPE must be used to prevent exposure to bloodborne pathogens and include the items covered in the following sections.

Gloves

OSHA and the CDC mandate that gloves be worn at all times when collecting blood samples. Gloves must be changed and hands washed between patients. The wearing of gloves does not eliminate the need for hand sanitizing. Alcohol-based hand sanitizers are an accepted substitute for hand washing except when the hands are visibly contaminated or the blood collector has been in an isolation room in which the patient has been diagnosed with a *Clostridium difficile* infection.

 SAFETY TIP 1-2

Wearing artificial nails is prohibited because of the possible spread of infection.

TABLE 1-1 Transmission-Based Precautions Classifications

Type	Possible Conditions	PPE
Airborne	Tuberculosis, measles, chickenpox, herpes zoster/shingles, mumps, adenovirus	Standard Precautions Mask or respirator
Droplet	Infection with *Neisseria meningitides*, *Haemophilus* sp., pertussis/whooping cough, group A streptococcus, influenza, rhinovirus, scarlet fever, parvovirus B19, respiratory syncytial virus, and diphtheria	Standard Precautions Mask
Contact	*Clostridium difficile*, rotavirus, draining wounds, antibiotic-resistant infections, scabies, impetigo, herpes simplex, respiratory syncytial virus, and herpes zoster	Standard Precautions Gown and gloves

PPE = personal protective equipment
Reproduced with permission from Strasinger, S.K., and Di Lorenzo, M.S.: The Phlebotomy Textbook, ed. 3. Philadelphia, F.A. Davis, 2011.

BOX 1-3 **Transmission Prevention Guidelines for Blood Collectors**

- Wear appropriate PPE.
- Change gloves between patients.
- Sanitize hands after removing gloves.
- Dispose of biohazardous material in designated containers.
- Properly dispose of sharps in puncture-resistant containers.
- Do not recap needles.
- Do not activate needle safety device using both hands.
- Follow institutional protocol governing working during personal illness.
- Maintain personal immunizations.
- Decontaminate work areas and equipment.
- Do not centrifuge uncapped tubes.
- Do not eat, drink, smoke, or apply cosmetics in the work area.

Reproduced with permission from Strasinger, S.K., and Di Lorenzo, M.S.: The Phlebotomy Textbook, ed. 3. Philadelphia, F.A. Davis, 2011.

Gowns

Gowns or laboratory coats are recommended apparel. Blood collectors should wear laboratory coats with knitted cuffs and pull the gloves over the cuffs to cover exposed skin. Blood sprays resulting from venipuncture or dermal puncture are likely to occur from the fingers to the elbows and from the collarbone to the waist.

Masks, Goggles, and Face Shields

Masks are worn to protect against inhalation of droplets containing microorganisms from infective patients. Masks, goggles, and face shields are used to protect the mucous membranes of the mouth, nose, and eyes from splashing of blood or body substances.

Respirators

An individually fitted N95 respirator should be used for patients with suspected tuberculosis.

Sharps Hazards

Most bloodborne pathogen exposures associated with blood collection occur as a result of accidental puncture with a contaminated needle or lancet. A major significant exposure occurs when a deep puncture is caused by a needle that has been used to collect blood. Therefore, strict adherence to all safety precautions is essential. The Needlestick Safety and Prevention Act of 2002 requires employers to provide sharps with engineered sharps injury protection features and to solicit employee input in selecting and reviewing these devices (http://www.osha.gov/SLTC/bloodbornepathogens) **(Box 1-4).**

 SAFETY TIP 1-3

Never recap needles and always discard them in puncture-resistant containers located close to the patient.

A variety of safety devices for needle disposal and also a variety of protective needle sheaths are available. (See Chapter 2, "Venipuncture Equipment.") It is extremely important that personnel become totally familiar with the use of these safety devices. Many accidental punctures occur because personnel do not know how to properly use the available safety devices.

Blood collected using a syringe must be transferred to the appropriate evacuated tubes using a blood transfer device. Removing the rubber stopper, adding the blood from the syringe, and restoppering the tube is not recommended because aerosols are produced and tubes are not as tightly stoppered for transport.

Needles with safety devices activated, syringes with needles attached, winged blood collections sets, and holders with needles attached are disposed of directly into puncture-resistant containers.

Sample Processing

Personnel working in off-site facilities or physicians' offices may be required to perform initial sample processing, such as centrifugation and separation of serum or plasma from blood cells. Centrifugation of uncapped tubes produces potentially harmful aerosols. Tubes must be carefully balanced in the centrifuge to prevent breakage, and the centrifuge lid must remain closed during operation to protect workers from exposure to blood and glass should a breakage occur. To prevent aerosol exposure when removing stoppers from evacuated tubes, first cover the stopper with gauze and then twist rather than "pop" off. Aerosols are also produced when specimens are poured rather than pipetted during transfer between

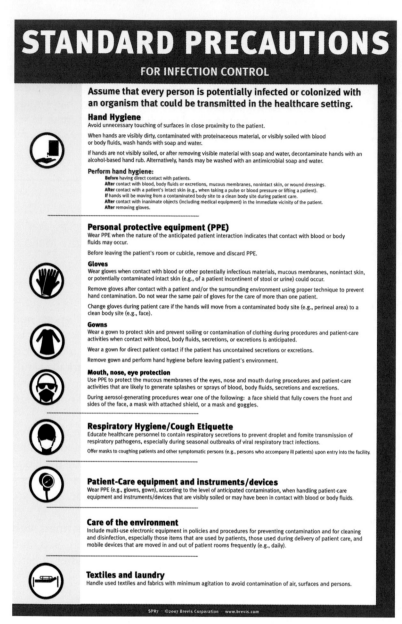

FIGURE 1-2 Standard Precautions. *(Reproduced with permission from Strasinger, S.K., and Di Lorenzo, M.S.: The Phlebotomy Textbook, ed. 3. Philadelphia, F.A. Davis, 2011.)*

tubes. A Plexiglas shield should be used when taking an **aliquot** from a sample.

Sample Transport

Samples must be packaged correctly and carefully for transport **(Fig. 1-3).** Samples for local transport should be placed in securely closed, leak-proof primary containers (tubes and screw-top containers). The primary containers are enclosed in a secondary leakproof container with sufficient absorbent material present to separate the samples and absorb the contents of the primary containers in case of leakage or breakage. Containers should be labeled as biohazardous. Samples that are transported via a pneumatic tube system must be placed in a labeled biohazard plastic bag and correctly cushioned to avoid breakage of the tube or hemolysis of the blood.

Postexposure Prophylaxis

Any accidental exposure to blood through needlestick, mucous membranes, or nonintact skin must be reported to a supervisor, and a confidential medical examination must be started immediately. Evaluation of the incident must begin immediately to ensure appropriate PEP is initiated within 24 hours. Procedures are explained in **Box 1-5.**

BOX 1-4 Components of the OSHA Bloodborne Pathogen Standard

ENGINEERING CONTROLS

1. Providing sharps disposal containers and needles with safety devices.
2. Requiring discarding of needles with the safety device activated and the holder attached.
3. Labeling all biohazardous materials and containers.

WORK PRACTICE CONTROLS

1. Requiring all employees to practice standard precautions.
2. Prohibiting eating, drinking, smoking, and applying cosmetics in the work area.
3. Establishing a daily work surface disinfection protocol.

PERSONAL PROTECTIVE EQUIPMENT

1. Providing laboratory coats, gowns, face shields, and gloves to employees and laundry facilities for nondisposable protective clothing.

MEDICAL

1. Providing immunization for the hepatitis B virus free of charge.
2. Providing medical follow-up to employees who have been accidentally exposed to bloodborne pathogens.

DOCUMENTATION

1. Documenting annual training of employees in safety standards.
2. Documenting evaluations and implementation of safer needle devices.
3. Involving employees in the selection and evaluation of new devices and maintaining a list of those employees and the evaluations.
4. Maintaining a sharps injury log including the type and brand of safety device, location and description of the incident, and confidential employee follow-up.

Reproduced with permission from Strasinger, S.K., and Di Lorenzo, M.S.: The Phlebotomy Textbook, ed. 3. Philadelphia, F.A. Davis, 2011.

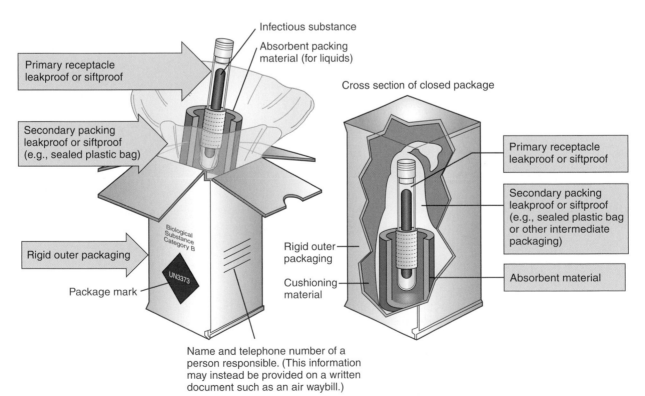

FIGURE 1-3 Packing and labeling of Category B infectious substances. *(Reproduced with permission from Strasinger, S.K., and Di Lorenzo, M.S.: The Phlebotomy Textbook, ed. 3. Philadelphia, F.A. Davis, 2011. Redrawn from Pipeline and Hazardous Materials Safety Administration, U.S. Department of Transportation.)*

BOX 1-5   Postexposure Prophylaxis

1. Draw a baseline blood sample from the employee and test it for HBV, HCV, and HIV.
2. If possible, identify the source patient, collect a blood sample, and test it for HBV, HCV, and HIV. Patients must usually give informed consent for these tests, and they do not become part of the patient's record. In some states, a physician's order or court order can replace patient consent because a needlestick is considered a significant exposure.
3. Testing must be completed within 24 hours for maximum benefit from PEP.

Source patient tests positive for HIV:

1. Employee is counseled about receiving PEP using zidovudine (ZDV) and one or two additional anti-HIV medications.
2. Medications are started within 24 hours.

3. Employee is retested at intervals of 6 weeks, 12 weeks, and 6 months.
4. Additional evaluation and counseling are needed if the source patient is unidentified or untested.

Source patient tests positive for HBV:

1. Unvaccinated employees can be given hepatitis B immune globulin (HBIg) and HBV vaccine.
2. Vaccinated employees are tested for immunity and receive PEP, if necessary.

Source patient tests positive for HCV:

1. No PEP is available.
2. Employee is monitored for early detection of HCV infection and treated appropriately.

Reproduced with permission from Strasinger, S.K., and Di Lorenzo, M.S.: The Phlebotomy Textbook, ed. 3. Philadelphia, F.A. Davis, 2011.

QUALITY MANAGEMENT

Laboratory quality management is designed to guarantee quality patient care by ensuring accurate and reliable test results in an appropriate and timely manner. As can be seen from this brief introduction, many factors related to blood collection can affect laboratory quality management. These factors are covered in detail in the following chapters. In addition, remember that laboratory personnel are available to answer questions and should be consulted whenever necessary.

BIBLIOGRAPHY

Clinical Laboratory Improvement Amendments. http://www.cdc.gov/clia/

CLSI: *Protection of Laboratory Workers From Occupational Acquired Infections*, ed. 4. Approved Guideline, M29-A4. Wayne, PA, CLSI, 2014.

INTERNET RESOURCES

http://www.cdc.gov/niosh/topics/bbp

http://www.clsi.org

http://www.fda.gov

http://www.osha.gov

http://www.cdc.gov/mmwr

http://www.osha.gov/SLTC/bloodbornepathogens

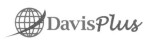 **DavisPlus**   For additional material, please visit http://davisplus.fadavis.com.

REVIEW QUESTIONS

1. All of the following are responsibilities of the blood collector except:
   a. Correct patient identification
   b. Quality of the sample
   c. Test results within normal limits
   d. Correct timing for the collection of the sample

2. The recommended disinfectant for cleaning blood and body fluid contamination is:
   a. Antibacterial soap
   b. Sodium hypochlorite
   c. Isopropyl alcohol
   d. Chlorhexidine gluconate

3. Failure to become familiar with needle disposal equipment can result in:
   a. Hemolyzed samples
   b. Failure to obtain the sample
   c. A clotted anticoagulated sample
   d. An accidental needlestick

4. OSHA requires employers of health-care workers to provide employees with all of the following except:
   a. Personal protective equipment
   b. HCV immunizations
   c. HBV immunizations
   d. Needles with safety devices

5. In the chain of infection, the susceptible host can also become the:
   a. Portal of entry
   b. Portal of exit
   c. Reservoir
   d. Means of transmission

6. All of the following are recognized as accrediting agencies by the Centers for Medicare & Medicaid Services except the:
   a. College of American Pathologists
   b. Clinical Laboratory Standards Institute
   c. The Joint Commission
   d. Commission on Laboratory Accreditation

7. What is the purpose of always closing the centrifuge lid when in use?
   a. Protection of the sample from light rays
   b. Protection of the worker from broken glass
   c. Protection of the sample from hemolysis
   d. Protection of the centrifuge's light

8. Guaranteeing accurate test results, timely delivery of samples to the laboratory, and quality patient care are all examples of:
   a. Sample processing
   b. OSHA requirements
   c. Quality management
   d. CLIA-waived testing

9. The laboratory regulation agency that is made up of laboratory, industry, and government personnel is the:
   a. CLSI
   b. CAP
   c. COLA
   d. CMS

10. A phlebotomy error that could lead to the death of a patient is:
    a. Failure to collect the sample on time
    b. Misidentifying the patient
    c. Collecting the sample in the wrong tube
    d. Failure to correctly centrifuge the sample

FOR FURTHER STUDY

1. Describe what the CLIA is and explain the three levels of laboratory testing.

2. Using the chain of infection, answer the following questions:
   a. What safety measure is shown to break the chain in four locations?
   b. In what area could reusing the same needle for a second puncture cause infection?
   c. In what area could failure to correctly dispose of the contaminated needle cause infection?

3. Give an example of an error in blood collection that relates to each of the regulations covered in this chapter.
   a. Standard precautions
   b. HIPAA
   c. OSHA Bloodborne Pathogen Standard
   d. Postexposure prophylaxis

CASE STUDY 1

Marsha is learning to perform phlebotomy. It is her first day collecting blood from patients. Marsha successfully performs the venipuncture; however, while attempting to recap the needle she accidentally punctures her finger. Marsha looks at the requisition again and notes that the patient is being tested for HIV.

1. What is it most important for Marsha to do?

2. How could this accident have been avoided?

3. If the patient tests positive for HIV, what should be done for Marsha?

CASE STUDY 2

When working in a physician's office, Jerry was required to perform sample processing before a sample was sent to the laboratory. The laboratory may require serum or plasma.

1. State the requirements for centrifuging a sample.

2. After centrifuging, how should the serum or plasma be removed from the tube?

3. How should the specimen be packaged for transport to the laboratory?

Venipuncture Equipment

LEARNING OBJECTIVES

Upon completion of this chapter, the reader will be able to:

2.1 Describe the basic function of hemostasis and coagulation.

2.2 Differentiate between the different types of blood samples.

2.3 Explain the actions of anticoagulants to prevent blood coagulation.

2.4 Discuss the current venipuncture collection materials and safety equipment.

2.5 Identify the types of evacuated tubes by color code, additive, and purpose.

2.6 List the correct order of draw for the various types of blood collection tubes.

2.7 Describe the quality control of venipuncture equipment.

Anticoagulant Substance that prevents blood from clotting

Antiglycolytic Agent Substance that prevents the breakdown of glucose

Antiseptic A substance used to clean the skin from contamination by microorganisms

Bevel Area of the needle point that has been cut on a slant

Hemolyzed Destruction of red blood cells

Hemostasis Stoppage of blood flow from a damaged blood vessel

Holder Plastic apparatus that attaches to a multi-sample needle or winged blood collection

Hub The part of the needle that attaches to the syringe or blood collection holder

Hypodermic Needle Type of needle that attaches to a syringe

Icteric Appearing yellow because of the presence of increased bilirubin

Lipemic Appearing cloudy white from increased lipids

Lumen Cavity of an organ or tube, such as a blood vessel or a needle

Multi-sample Needle Type of needle that attaches to a holder to collect multiple blood collection tubes

Plasma Liquid portion of unclotted or anticoagulated blood that contains fibrinogen

Plasma Separator Tube (PST) Type of collection tube that contains a polymer gel that separates blood cells from the plasma when centrifuged

Serum Liquid portion that remains after clotted blood has been centrifuged and separated that does not contain fibrinogen

Serum Separator Tube (SST) Type of collection tube that contains a polymer gel that separates the blood cells from the serum when centrifuged

Winged Blood Collection Set Type of needle and tubing apparatus with plastic wings attached that can connect to a holder or syringe

INTRODUCTION

Considering the many types of blood specimens that may be required for laboratory testing and the risks to both patients and health-care personnel associated with blood collection, it is understandable that a considerable amount of equipment is required for the procedure.

This chapter describes coagulation and **hemostasis,** the types of specimens, various blood collection systems, collection tubes, order of draw, safety disposal systems, and other required supplies necessary for efficient blood collection. **Box 2-1** lists routine venipuncture equipment.

COAGULATION AND HEMOSTASIS

Hemostasis is the process of forming a blood clot to stop the leakage of blood when injury to a blood vessel occurs and lysing the clot when the injury has been repaired. A complex coagulation mechanism that involves blood vessels, platelets, and the coagulation factors maintains hemostasis. A basic understanding of coagulation can be obtained by dividing the process into four stages as shown in **Figures 2-1** through **2-4.** The amount of time the blood takes to clot often depends on the type of blood vessel that has been punctured.

BOX 2-1 Routine Venipuncture Equipment

Phlebotomy collection tray
Evacuated tube system holders
Syringes
Winged blood collection sets
Needles
Needle disposal sharps containers
Evacuated collection tubes
Transfer devices
Tourniquets
Gloves
70 percent isopropyl alcohol, iodine swabs, chlorhexidine gluconate swabs
2 × 2 gauze pads
Bandages
Slides
Antimicrobial hand gel
Marking pen

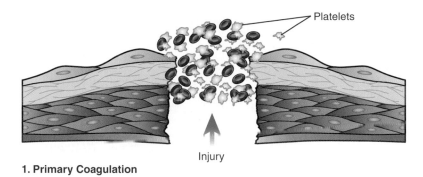

FIGURE 2-1 Stage 1 of the coagulation cascade. *(Reproduced with permission from Strasinger, S.K., and Di Lorenzo, M.S.: The Phlebotomy Textbook, ed. 3. Philadelphia, F.A. Davis, 2011.)*

1. Primary Coagulation

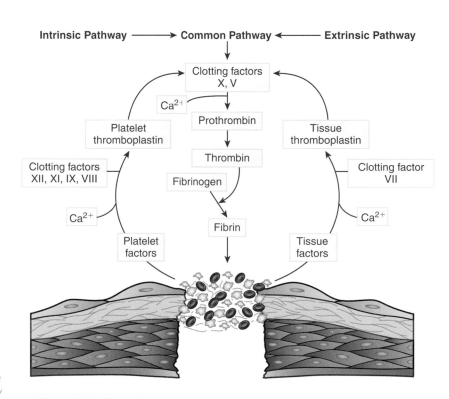

FIGURE 2-2 Stage 2 of the coagulation cascade. *(Reproduced with permission from Strasinger, S.K., and Di Lorenzo, M.S.: The Phlebotomy Textbook, ed. 3. Philadelphia, F.A. Davis, 2011.)*

2. Coagulation Cascade

TECHNICAL TIP 2-1

The activated partial thromboplastin time and the activated clotting time tests evaluate the intrinsic pathway and monitor heparin therapy. The prothrombin time test evaluates the extrinsic pathway and monitors Coumadin therapy.

TYPES OF BLOOD SAMPLES

Arterial Blood

Arterial blood is highly oxygenated and a bright red color that is pumped away from the heart to the capillaries. Pressure must be applied to the site for 3 to 5 minutes to stop the bleeding because of the increased blood flow. Arterial blood is the required sample for arterial blood gas determinations. In the interest of patient safety, only specifically

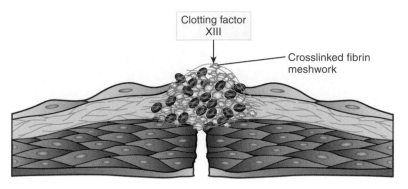

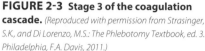

3. Fibrin Stabilizing, and Clot Retraction

FIGURE 2-3 **Stage 3 of the coagulation cascade.** *(Reproduced with permission from Strasinger, S.K., and Di Lorenzo, M.S.: The Phlebotomy Textbook, ed. 3. Philadelphia, F.A. Davis, 2011.)*

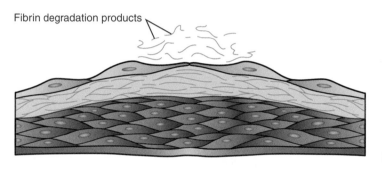

4. Fibrinolysis

FIGURE 2-4 **Stage 4 of the coagulation cascade.** *(Reproduced with permission from Strasinger, S.K., and Di Lorenzo, M.S.: The Phlebotomy Textbook, ed. 3. Philadelphia, F.A. Davis, 2011.)*

trained personnel may perform arterial punctures. Arterial blood also may be collected from central lines.

Venous Blood

Venous blood is obtained from veins and has a lower pressure that stops bleeding more quickly. Veins have one-way valves to keep blood flowing in one direction as the blood flows through the veins by skeletal muscle contraction. It is a dark red color because of the low levels of oxygen and high levels of carbon dioxide and waste products. Venous blood is the sample of choice for clinical laboratory testing because venipuncture samples provide more consistent and reliable test results. Reference ranges for laboratory tests are determined from venous blood.

Capillary Blood

Capillary blood is a mixture of arterial and venous blood and is collected by dermal puncture. Bleeding is controlled with slight pressure to the site. When properly collected, capillary blood is suitable for many laboratory tests, but reference ranges may differ from those of venous blood. Therefore, requisition forms should indicate whether the sample is arterial or capillary blood.

TYPES OF SPECIMENS

The laboratory refers to blood specimens primarily in terms of whole blood, **plasma,** and **serum.** A whole blood sample contains erythrocytes, leukocytes, and platelets suspended in plasma and essentially represent blood as it circulates through the body. Tests related to blood cells, such as the complete blood count (CBC) and blood typing, are performed on whole blood.

The majority of laboratory tests are performed on the liquid portion of blood (plasma or serum), which contains substances such as proteins, enzymes, organic and inorganic chemicals, and antibodies. Plasma is the liquid portion of blood that has not clotted; serum is the liquid portion remaining after clotting has occurred. Plasma is often defined as the liquid portion of blood that contains fibrinogen and other clotting factors, and serum as the liquid portion that does not contain fibrinogen and other clotting factors. Both serum and plasma are obtained by centrifugation of clotted or unclotted samples, which separates the cellular elements from the liquid portion **(Fig. 2-5).** The presence or absence of **anticoagulants** in the tubes into which blood samples are placed determines the type of

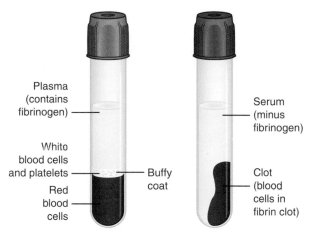

FIGURE 2-5 **Differences between plasma and serum.** *(Reproduced with permission from Strasinger, S.K., and Di Lorenzo, M.S.: The Phlebotomy Textbook, ed. 3. Philadelphia, F.A. Davis, 2011.)*

specimen available for testing. Whole blood and plasma require an anticoagulant to prevent clot formation. Serum is obtained from tubes that do not contain an anticoagulant.

Collection tubes contain a variety of anticoagulants, the chemical content of which must be considered in conjunction with the laboratory test requested. As shown in **Figure 2-6,** anticoagulants prevent coagulation by two different mechanisms. The anticoagulants dipotassium and tripotassium ethylenediaminetetraacetic acid (EDTA), sodium citrate, sodium polyanethol sulfonate (SPS), and potassium oxalate bind calcium, which is required by the coagulation cascade. Heparin in the form of sodium, ammonium, or lithium heparin inhibits the formation of thrombin that is required to convert fibrinogen into a fibrin clot.

With the obvious exception of coagulation tests, many laboratory tests can be performed on either serum or plasma. However, the anticoagulant composition and method of action must be considered when tests are to be run on plasma. For example, an EDTA tube cannot be used when a plasma calcium level is requested, because the plasma calcium will be bound to the EDTA, resulting in falsely decreased values. Reference ranges of some analytes also differ between serum and plasma. Laboratory protocols for sample collection specify the type of tube to be used. These protocols have been designed to ensure that the most representative test results are obtained, and they must be followed.

Normal serum and plasma appear clear and pale yellow. Variations in the normal appearance can indicate that certain test results may be adversely affected **(Fig. 2-7).**

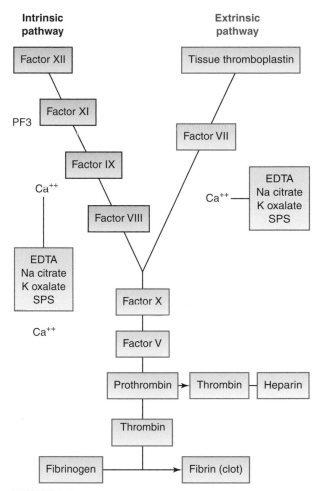

FIGURE 2-6 **The role of anticoagulants in the coagulation cascade.** *(Reproduced with permission from Strasinger, S.K., and Di Lorenzo, M.S.: The Phlebotomy Textbook, ed. 3. Philadelphia, F.A. Davis, 2011.)*

Examples of abnormal appearance that are discussed in more detail in later chapters include:

- **Hemolyzed**—Pink to red color, indicating red blood cell destruction **(Fig. 2-8)**
- **Icteric**—Dark yellow color, indicating the presence of increased bilirubin
- **Lipemic**—Cloudy, milky appearance, indicating the presence of increased lipids

ORGANIZATION OF EQUIPMENT

An important key to successful blood collection is making sure that all the required equipment is conveniently present in the collection area. Trays designed to organize and transport collection equipment are available from several manufacturers **(Fig. 2-9).**

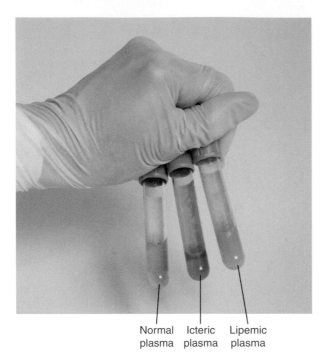

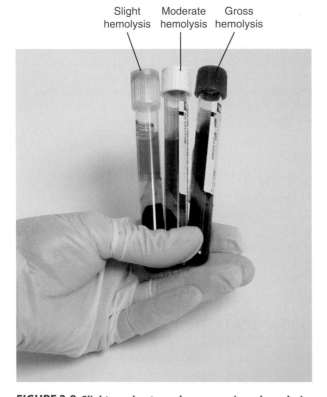

FIGURE 2-7 **Normal, incteric, and lipemic specimens.** *(Reproduced with permission from Strasinger, S.K., and Di Lorenzo, M.S.: The Phlebotomy Textbook, ed. 3. Philadelphia, F.A. Davis, 2011.)*

FIGURE 2-8 **Slight, moderate, and gross specimen hemolysis.** *(Reproduced with permission from Strasinger, S.K., and Di Lorenzo, M.S.: The Phlebotomy Textbook, ed. 3. Philadelphia, F.A. Davis, 2011.)*

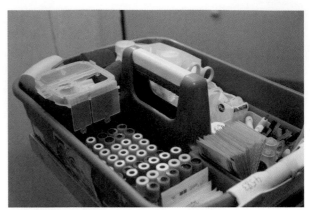

FIGURE 2-9 **Blood collection tray.** *(Reproduced with permission from Strasinger, S.K., and Di Lorenzo, M.S.: The Phlebotomy Textbook, ed. 3. Philadelphia, F.A. Davis, 2011.)*

Maintaining a well-equipped blood collection tray that the blood collector carries into the patient's room (with the exception of isolation rooms) is the ideal way to prevent unnecessary errors during blood collection. Place the tray on a solid surface, such as a nightstand and not on the patient's bed, where it can be knocked off. Trays should be emptied and disinfected on a weekly basis and more frequently if they become visibly soiled.

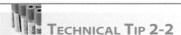 **TECHNICAL TIP 2-2**

A well-organized tray instills patient confidence.

Mobile phlebotomy workstations with swivel-caster wheels have replaced the traditional phlebotomy tray in some institutions. With the increased amounts of required equipment necessary for safe phlebotomy, these versatile mobile workstations can be configured to accommodate phlebotomy trays, hazardous waste containers, sharps containers, and storage drawers and shelves. The cart is designed to be wheeled around the hospital and up to the patient's bedside to eliminate placing equipment or a phlebotomy tray on the patient's bed **(Fig. 2-10).**

In outpatient settings, use a blood drawing chair with an attached or adjacently placed stand to hold equipment **(Fig. 2-11).** Drawing chairs have an armrest that locks in place in front of the patient to properly position the arm and to provide arm support and protect the patient from falling out of the chair if he or she

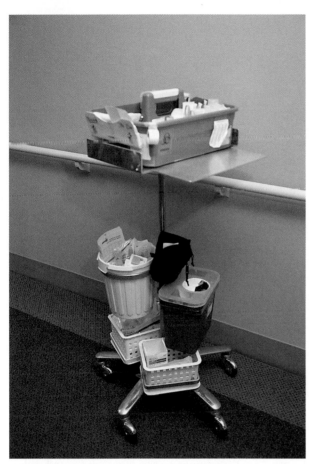

FIGURE 2-10 Mobile phlebotomy workstation. *(Reproduced with permission from Strasinger, S.K., and Di Lorenzo, M.S.: The Phlebotomy Textbook, ed. 3. Philadelphia, F.A. Davis, 2011.)*

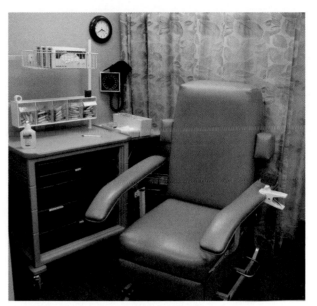

FIGURE 2-11 Phlebotomy drawing station, including a reclining chair. *(Reproduced with permission from Strasinger, S.K., and Di Lorenzo, M.S.: The Phlebotomy Textbook, ed. 3. Philadelphia, F.A. Davis, 2011.)*

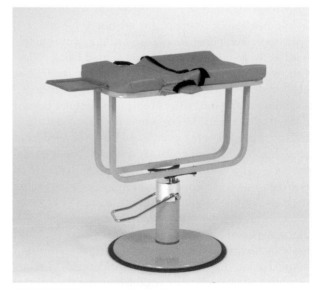

FIGURE 2-12 Infant cradle pad. *(Courtesy of Innovative Laboratory Acrylics, Inc., Brighton, MI.)*

faints. A reclining chair or bed should be available for special procedures or for patients who feel faint or ill. Infant cradle pads are available for collection of blood from an infant **(Fig. 2-12).**

Venipuncture can be performed using an evacuated tube system (ETS), a syringe system, or a winged blood collection set. Each of these systems requires its own unique equipment, which is discussed in the following sections. Supplies that are common to all procedures also are discussed.

EVACUATED TUBE SYSTEM (ETS)

The evacuated tube system (ETS) **(Fig. 2-13)** is the most frequently used method for performing venipuncture and is available from various manufacturers. Blood is collected directly into the evacuated tube, eliminating the need for transfer of samples and minimizing the risk of biohazard exposure. The evacuated tube system consists of a double-pointed needle with one point to puncture the patient's vein and the other point to puncture the tube stopper, a holder to hold the needle, and color-coded evacuated tubes.

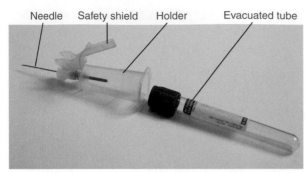

FIGURE 2-13 Evacuated tube system. *(Reproduced with permission from Strasinger, S.K., and Di Lorenzo, M.S.: The Phlebotomy Textbook, ed. 3. Philadelphia, F.A. Davis, 2011.)*

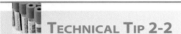

TECHNICAL TIP 2-2

It is recommended not to interchange evacuated tube system components from different manufacturers.

Needles

Sterile needles for venipuncture are disposable and used only once. Venipuncture needles include **multi-sample needles, hypodermic needles,** and **winged blood collection needles.** Multi-sample needles are packaged in sterile, twist-apart sealed shields that are color-coded according to the size of the needle and must not be used if the seal is broken. Multi-sample needles used with an ETS are threaded in the middle and have a **beveled** point at each end. The front end is used to enter the vein, and the back end is used to penetrate the rubber stopper of an evacuated tube. A retractable rubber sheath covers the back end of the needle to prevent leakage of blood as tubes are changed or removed. Syringe hypodermic needles and winged blood collection set needles are packaged individually in sterile packets. All needles consist of a beveled point, shaft, lumen, and **hub. Figure 2-14** shows the difference between the hypodermic (syringe needle) and the multi-sample needle structures. Needles should be visually examined for structural defects, such as no beveled points or bent shafts, immediately before use. Defective needles should not be used. Needles should never be recapped once the shield is removed regardless of whether they have or have not been used.

Needle size varies by both length and gauge and is indicated by color-coded caps. The needle gauge refers to the diameter of the needle: the lower the number, the larger the needle. Needles range from 20 to 23 gauge for

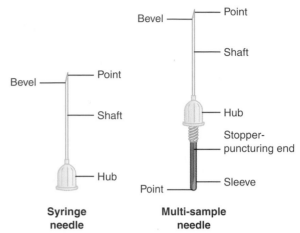

FIGURE 2-14 Needle structures. *(Reproduced with permission from Strasinger, S.K., and Di Lorenzo, M.S.: The Phlebotomy Textbook, ed. 3. Philadelphia, F.A. Davis, 2011.)*

venipuncture; however, the standard needles used with evacuated tubes are 21 or 22 gauge with a 1-inch or 1.5-inch length. Although a 20-gauge needle will allow blood to flow more quickly, it is not recommended for routine blood collection. Many patients are on blood thinners and the use of a 20-gauge needle can result in postpuncture bleeding and hematomas because of the larger opening in the vein. Children and patients with small veins may require 23-gauge needles with a 3/4-inch length. Small-volume partial-draw evacuated tubes should be used with small-gauge needles because a small-diameter needle with a large evacuated tube can cause hemolysis as the blood is being pulled through the small lumen of the needle by the vacuum in the collection tubes. Using 25-gauge needles is not recommended because of the longer time the needle is in the vein and the increased frequency of hemolysis. The small **lumen** size of the 25-gauge needle causes the tube to fill more slowly and microclots may form. Needles used to collect units of blood for transfusion are the larger, 16-gauge needles.

Many needles are equipped with safety shields and blunting devices. Safety features include devices that blunt the needle or retract the needle after use, or shields that cover the needle after use.

 SAFETY TIP 2-1

The Needlestick Safety and Prevention Act (Chapter 1) mandates the evaluation and implementation of safety devices.

Safety shields covering the needles have been introduced with the SafetyGlide blood collection system (Becton, Dickinson, Franklin Lakes, NJ). The blood collector pushes the movable shield along the cannula with the thumb to enclose the needle tip after venipuncture **(Fig. 2-15).**

The BD Vacutainer Eclipse blood collection needle uses a shield that the blood collector locks over the needle tip when the needle is removed from the vein **(Fig. 2-16, A and B).** It is available for both the ETS and syringe system.

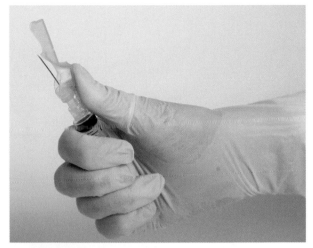

FIGURE 2-16B Eclipse blood collection needle for the syringe system. *(Reproduced with permission Strasinger, S.K., and Di Lorenzo, M.S.: The Phlebotomy Textbook, ed. 3. Philadelphia, F.A. Davis, 2011.)*

 SAFETY TIP 2-2

Always confirm an audible click is heard to verify that the safety shield is locked in place.

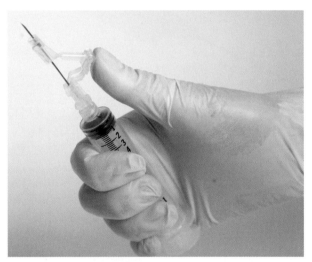

FIGURE 2-15 SafetyGlide blood collection assembly. *(Reproduced with permission from Strasinger, S.K., and Di Lorenzo, M.S.: The Phlebotomy Textbook, ed. 3. Philadelphia, F.A. Davis, 2011.)*

The Venipuncture Needle-Pro (Smiths Medical, St. Paul, MN) resheaths the needle by pressing the shield against a hard surface to click over the needle. It is connected to the holder for both the ETS system and attached to the needle for the syringe system **(Fig. 2-17, A, B, and C).**

 SAFETY TIP 2-3

The Venipuncture Needle-Pro safety shield must never be activated with the thumb to avoid an accidental needlestick.

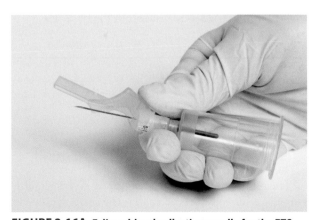

FIGURE 2-16A Eclipse blood collection needle for the ETS. *(Reproduced with permission from Strasinger, S.K., and Di Lorenzo, M.S.: The Phlebotomy Textbook, ed. 3. Philadelphia, F.A. Davis, 2011.)*

Self-blunting needles (Punctur-Guard by Gaven Medical, Vernon, CT) are available to provide additional protection against needlestick injuries by making the needle blunt before removal from the patient. A hollow, blunt inner needle is contained inside the standard needle. Before removing the needle from the patient's vein, an additional push on the final tube in the holder advances the internal blunt cannula past the sharp tip of the outer

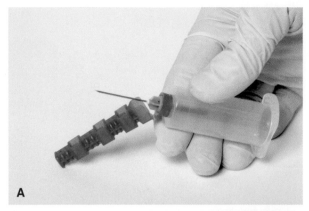

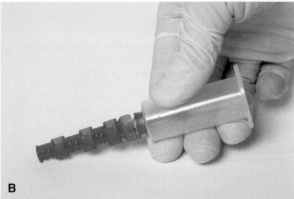

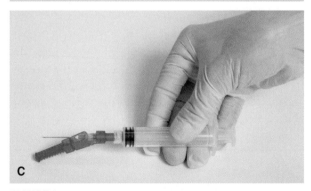

FIGURE 2-17 **Venipuncture Needle-Pro for the ETS.** *A,* **Activating shield on a hard surface.** *B,* **Shield fully engaged.** *C,* **Venipuncture Needle-Pro for the syringe system.** *(Reproduced with permission from Strasinger, S.K., and Di Lorenzo, M.S.: The Phlebotomy Textbook, ed. 3. Philadelphia, F.A. Davis, 2011.)*

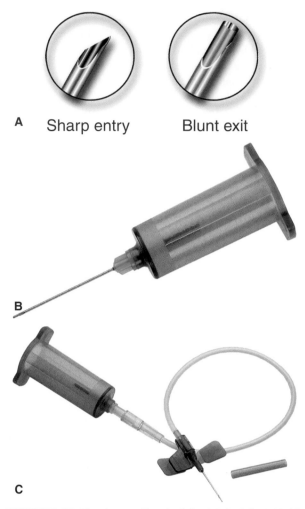

FIGURE 2-18 **Blunting needle principle.** *A,* **Principle.** *B,* **Multisample needle attached to a holder.** *C,* **Winged blood collection set.** *(Courtesy of Gaven Medical, Vernon, CT.)*

a sterile preattached multi-sample needle with safety shield. Various holders are shown in **Figure 2-19.**

⚠ **SAFETY TIP 2-4**

If the evacuated tube needle does not have a safety device, the tube holder must have one.

---

needle. The blunt cannula is hollow, allowing blood to continue to flow into the tube **(Fig. 2-18, A, B, and C).**

Needle Holders

Needle **holders** used with ETSs are made of clear, rigid plastic and are available with or without safety features. Complete units are available that include the holder and

The rubber-sheathed tube puncturing end of a multi-sample needle screws securely into the small opening at one end of the holder, and the evacuated blood collection tube is placed into the large opening at the opposite end of the holder. The first tube is partially advanced on

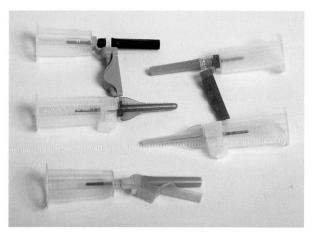

FIGURE 2-19 Various types of tube holders. *(Reproduced with permission from Strasinger, S.K., and Di Lorenzo, M.S.: The Phlebotomy Textbook, ed. 3. Philadelphia, F.A. Davis, 2011.)*

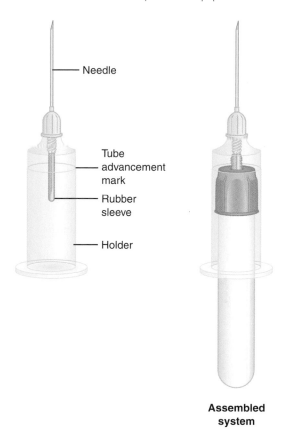

Needle

Tube advancement mark

Rubber sleeve

Holder

Assembled system

FIGURE 2-20 Diagram of a basic needle holder. *(Reproduced with permission from Strasinger, S.K., and Di Lorenzo, M.S.: The Phlebotomy Textbook, ed. 3. Philadelphia, F.A. Davis, 2011.)*

to the stopper-puncturing needle up to a designated mark on the holder. Pushing the tube beyond this point will prematurely release the tube's vacuum, making the tube unusable. The tube is fully advanced on to the end of the holder when the needle is in the vein. Blood will flow into the tube once the needle penetrates the stopper. The flared ends of the holder aid the blood collector during the changing of tubes in multiple-tube situations **(Fig. 2-20).** Tubes are removed with a slight twist to help disengage them from the needle.

 TECHNICAL TIP 2-4

Loss of tube vacuum is a primary cause of failure to obtain blood. The venipuncture can be performed before placing the tube on the needle. Practice both methods and choose the one with which you are most comfortable.

Several safety holders are available that include a protective shield that covers the needle after use or automatically retracts the needle into the holder after venipuncture **(Fig. 2-21).**

Venipuncture Needle-Pro (Smiths Medical, St. Paul, MN) uses a plastic shield attached by a hinge to the end of the evacuated tube holder. The shield hangs free during the venipuncture and when engaged against a hard surface, the needle is encapsulated by the shield. The entire device is discarded in the sharps container.

The ProGuard II safety needle holder (Covidien, Mansfield, MA) uses a one-handed method to manually retract the needle into the holder and a hinged cover locks in place to protect the back end that is open to the stopper-puncturing needle.

The VanishPoint tube holder (Retractable Technologies, Little Elm, TX) automatically retracts the needle by securely closing the end cap after the last tube has been removed while the needle is still in the patient's vein **(Fig. 2-22, A and B).**

The VACUETTE QuickShield Safety Tube Holder (Greiner Bio-One International AG, Kremsmunster, Austria) comes with a protective cap and is designed to use with VACUETTE multi-sample needles. The VACUETTE QuickShield Complete style includes both the holder and a sterile preattached needle. After completion of blood collection, the needle is removed from the patient's vein and the protective cap is pressed over the needle against a hard surface using a one-handed technique. The VACUETTE QuickShield Complete Plus system includes a holder and a VACUETTE® VISIO

BD One-Use holder

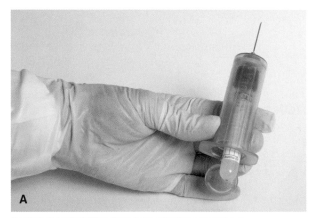

Venipuncture
Needle-Pro

VanishPoint

**FIGURE 2-21 Venipuncture Needle-Pro, VanishPoint, BD
holders.** *(Reproduced with permission from Strasinger, S.K., and Di Lorenzo, M.S.:
The Phlebotomy Textbook, ed. 3. Philadelphia, F.A. Davis, 2011.)*

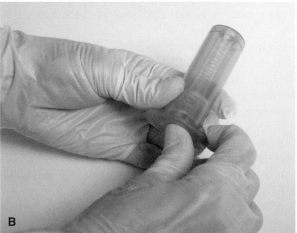

FIGURE 2-22 *A,* **VanishPoint tube holder before venipuncture.** *B,* **Tube removed, needle retracted and sealed after
venipuncture.** *(Reproduced with permission from Strasinger, S.K., and Di
Lorenzo, M.S.: The Phlebotomy Textbook, ed. 3. Philadelphia, F.A. Davis, 2011.)*

PLUS multi-sample needle with a see-through hub. In
this combination, a "flash" is observed that confirms
penetration of the vein.

The BD Vacutainer® Passive Shielding Blood Collection Needle (Becton, Dickinson) and the VAC-
UETTE Premium Safety Needle System (Greiner
Bio-One) are the new generation of safety devices. The
systems include a preassembled multi-sample needle with
safety device and holder. In both systems, the insertion
of the first tube into the holder releases the safety shield,
which then rests against the patient's skin. As the needle
is removed from the vein after blood collection, a spring
in the holder causes the safety shield to automatically
move forward to cover the needle. An advantage to these
systems is that the needle is immediately covered when
the needle moves out of the vein as the result of an unexpected move by the patient. Both systems have a safety
shield indicator arrow that judges the depth of needle insertion. The holders have a flat side to lie against the skin
for shallow angle of needle entry **(Fig. 2-23).**

The S-Monovette Blood Collection System (Sarstedt, Inc., Newton, NC) is an enclosed multi-sampling

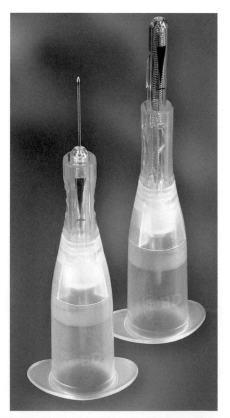

**FIGURE 2-23 BD Vacutainer Passive Shielding Blood Collec-
tion Needle.** *(Courtesy of Becton, Dickinson and Company.)*

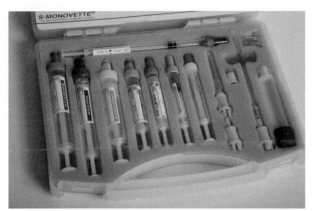

FIGURE 2-24 S-Monovette Blood Collection System (Sarstedt, Inc., Newton, NC). *(Reproduced with permission from Strasinger, S.K., and Di Lorenzo, M.S.: The Phlebotomy Textbook, ed. 3. Philadelphia, F.A. Davis, 2011.)*

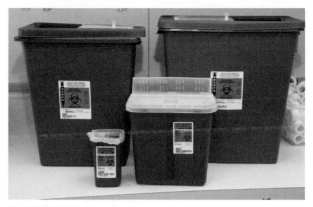

FIGURE 2-25 Sharps disposal containers. *(Reproduced with permission from Strasinger, S.K., and Di Lorenzo, M.S.: The Phlebotomy Textbook, ed. 3. Philadelphia, F.A. Davis, 2011.)*

blood collection system that includes the blood collection tube and collection device. Blood is collected using either manual aspiration or vacuum principle of collection with multi-sampling needles with preassembled holders and needle-protection devices. The aspiration technique is similar to a syringe draw. The system uses plastic tubes with screw caps **(Fig. 2-24).**

Collection Tubes

The collection tubes used with the ETS **(Fig. 2-26, A and B)** are available in a variety of sizes and volumes ranging from 1.8 to 15 mL. The amount of blood collected is determined by the size of the tube and the amount of vacuum present. Both glass and plastic tubes are available but glass tubes are less desirable because

 SAFETY TIP 2-5

To prevent accidental punctures from contaminated needles, become thoroughly familiar with the operation of your needle safety system before performing blood collection.

Needle Disposal Systems

Needles must always be placed in rigid, puncture-resistant, leakproof disposable containers labeled BIOHAZARD that are easily sealed when full. Syringes with the needles attached, winged blood collection sets, and holders with needles attached are disposed of directly into puncture-resistant containers **(Fig. 2-25).** *Under no circumstances should a needle be manually recapped.*

 SAFETY TIP 2-6

Sharps containers should be filled only to the designated mark and never overfilled.

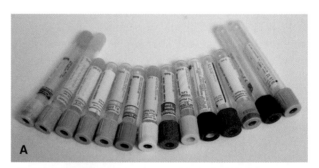

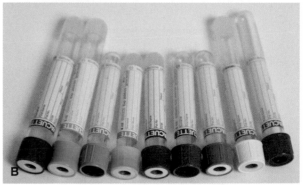

FIGURE 2-26 Evacuated tubes. *A,* BD Vacutainer tubes (Becton, Dickinson, Franklin Lakes, NJ). *B,* VACUETTE evacuated tubes (Greiner Bio-One, Monroe, NC). *(Reproduced with permission from Strasinger, S.K., and Di Lorenzo, M.S.: The Phlebotomy Textbook, ed. 3. Philadelphia, F.A. Davis, 2011.)*

of the risk of breakage and exposure to bloodborne pathogens. The tubes are labeled with the type of anticoagulant or additive, the draw volume, and the expiration date. Two types of color-coded tops are available. Evacuated tubes have color-coded rubber stoppers or plastic shields covering the rubber stoppers (Becton, Dickinson Hemogard Vacutainer System, Franklin Lakes, NJ) to indicate the presence or absence of an additive or anticoagulant in the tube. The color-coding is generally universal; however, it may vary slightly by manufacturer, and describes the type of tube to use for sample collection, for example, "Draw one red stopper and one light blue stopper tube." This reference to tube color is found on most computer-generated requisition forms. Each laboratory department has specific specimen requirements for the analysis of particular blood constituents.

As shown in **Figure 2-27,** evacuated tubes have thick rubber stoppers with a thinner central area to allow puncture by the needle. Tubes may have a color-coded plastic safety shield covering the stopper to provide additional protection against blood splatter (BD Hemogard Vacutainer System) when stoppers are removed. Tubes are designed to be placed on the laboratory instrument and can be bar coded for identification and sampled directly by means of an instrument probe that pierces the stopper.

Evacuated tubes fill automatically because a premeasured vacuum is present in the tube. This causes some tubes to fill almost to the top, whereas other tubes fill only partially. BD partial-draw tubes are distinguished from regular tubes by translucent-colored Hemogard closures in the same color as regular tubes. VACUETTE partial-draw tubes are indicated by a white ring in the cap color. The draw volume is written on the tube label. When a tube has lost its vacuum, it cannot fill to the correct level. Loss of vacuum can be caused by dropping the tube, opening the tube, improper storage, manufacturer error, using the tube past its expiration date, prematurely advancing the tube on to the stopper-puncturing needle in the holder, or pulling the needle bevel out of the skin during venipuncture. Tubes are sterile and silicone coated to prevent cells from adhering to the wall of the tube, thereby decreasing hemolysis.

Tests requiring whole blood or plasma are collected in tubes containing an anticoagulant such as potassium oxalate, sodium citrate, EDTA, and heparin. Different types of anticoagulants are required for specific tests. All tubes containing an anticoagulant must be gently inverted three to eight times (depending on the type of tube) immediately after collection to mix the contents and to avoid microclot formation. Tubes containing an anticoagulant must be completely filled to the designated volume draw. If the blood-to-anticoagulant ratio is incorrect, test results may be erroneous. Partial-draw collection tubes should be used when a short draw is anticipated. Other additives present in evacuated tubes are used as preservatives and clot activators. Tubes containing additives also must be gently mixed to ensure effectiveness. Blood collected in a tube containing an anticoagulant or additive cannot be transferred into a tube containing a different anticoagulant or additive. **(See Fig. 2-28.)**

 TECHNICAL TIP 2-5

Shaking an anticoagulated tube rather than gently inverting the tube may cause hemolysis and the sample will be rejected.

 TECHNICAL TIP 2-6

Observing an air bubble moving through the tube from top to bottom during inversion ensures proper mixing.

 TECHNICAL TIP 2-7

For anticoagulants to totally prevent clotting, samples must be thoroughly mixed immediately following collection.

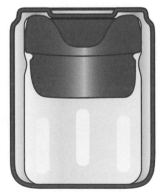

FIGURE 2-27 Cut-away view of a vacuum tube stopper (Hemogard closure). *(Adapted from product literature, Becton, Dickinson, Franklin Lakes, NJ. Reproduced with permission from Strasinger, S.K., and Di Lorenzo, M.S.: The Phlebotomy Textbook, ed. 3. Philadelphia, F.A. Davis, 2011.)*

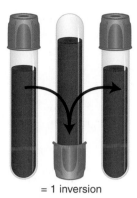

= 1 inversion

FIGURE 2-28 Evacuated tube inversion. *(Reproduced with permission from Strasinger, S.K., and Di Lorenzo, M.S.: Phlebotomy Notes: Pocket Guide to Blood Collection. Philadelphia, F.A. Davis, 2013.)*

 SAFETY TIP 2-7

Removing the stoppers from evacuated tubes can be hazardous because an aerosol of blood can be produced if the stopper is quickly "popped off." Stopper should be covered with a gauze pad and slowly loosened with the opening facing away from the body.

Color-Coding of Tubes

Lavender (Purple) Top

Lavender stopper tubes contain the anticoagulant EDTA in the form of liquid tripotassium (K_3EDTA) (glass) or spray-coated dipotassium ethylenediaminetetraacetic acid (K_2EDTA) (plastic). Coagulation is prevented by the binding of calcium in the sample to sites on the large EDTA molecule, thereby preventing the participation of the calcium in the coagulation cascade **(see Fig. 2-6).** Lavender stopper tubes should be gently inverted eight times for adequate mixing. For hematology procedures that require whole blood, such as the CBC, K_2EDTA is the anticoagulant of choice because it maintains cellular integrity better than do other anticoagulants, inhibits platelet clumping, and does not interfere with routine staining procedures. In an underfilled EDTA tube, the excess anticoagulant may shrink red blood cells and decrease the hematocrit level, red blood cell indices, and erythrocyte sedimentation rate (ESR) rates. However, the tubes can be submitted to the laboratory for evaluation if necessary. The Clinical and Laboratory Standards Institute (CLSI) recommends K_2EDTA for hematology tests because liquid K_3EDTA dilutes the sample and results in lower results. K_2EDTA tubes may be used for immunohematology testing and blood donor screening. As shown in Figure 2-6, lavender stopper tubes cannot be used for coagulation studies because EDTA interferes with factor V and the thrombin-fibrinogen reaction.

Pink Top

Pink stopper tubes also contain a spray-coated K_2EDTA anticoagulant and are used specifically for blood bank in some facilities. Using a designated tube for a blood bank is believed to help prevent testing of samples from the wrong patient. The tubes are designed with special labels for patient information required by the American Association of Blood Banks (AABB). Tubes should be inverted eight times.

White Top

White stopper tubes containing a spray-coated K_2EDTA anticoagulant and a separation gel are called plasma preparation tubes (PPT). This differentiates them from plasma separator tubes that contain heparin as the anticoagulant. White stopper tubes are primarily used for molecular diagnostics test methods but can be used for myocardial infarction (MI) panels and ammonia levels, depending on the test methodology and instrumentation. Greiner Bio-One VACUETTE K_2EDTA tubes with gel have a lavender stopper with a yellow ring. Tubes should be inverted eight times.

Light Blue Top

Light blue stopper tubes contain the anticoagulant sodium citrate, which also prevents coagulation by binding calcium. Centrifugation of the anticoagulated light blue stopper tubes provides the plasma used for coagulation tests. Sodium citrate (3.2 or 3.8 percent) is the required anticoagulant for coagulation studies because it preserves the labile coagulation factors. Tubes should be gently inverted three to four times.

Special glass CTAD light blue stopper tubes contain citrate, theophylline, adenosine, and dipyridamole and are used for selected platelet function assays. Greiner Bio-One VACUETTE CTAD tubes have blue stoppers with a yellow ring.

 TECHNICAL TIP 2-8

Overmixing a light blue stopper tube can activate platelets and produce erroneous coagulation test results.

The ratio of blood to liquid sodium citrate is critical and should be 9:1 (example: 4.5 mL blood and 0.5 mL sodium citrate). This tube requires a full draw to prevent dilution of coagulation factors. When drawing coagulation tests on patients with polycythemia or hematocrit readings more than 55 percent, the amount of anticoagulant must be decreased to maintain the 9:1 ratio, because the lower volume of plasma in these patients will be diluted by the standard volume of sodium citrate. Likewise, the amount of anticoagulant must be increased for severely anemic patients because of the larger amount of plasma. The laboratory should be consulted to provide tubes with the appropriate amount of anticoagulant.

TECHNICAL TIP 2-9

The laboratory always rejects incompletely filled light blue stopper tubes.

A special dark blue stopper tube containing thrombin and a soybean trypsin inhibitor is used when drawing blood for determinations of certain fibrin degradation products.

TECHNICAL TIP 2-10

Underfilled sodium citrate tubes will have an incorrect anticoagulant-to-blood ratio, which can cause a falsely lengthened APTT result.

TECHNICAL TIP 2-11

To maintain the correct blood-to-anticoagulant ratio for the blue stopper tube when using a winged blood collection set, a discard tube must be drawn prior to the collection tube to prime the line.

Black Top

Black stopper tubes containing sodium citrate are used for Westergren erythrocyte sedimentation rate determination (ESR). They differ from light blue stopper tubes in that they provide a ratio of blood to liquid anticoagulant of 4:1 Specially designed ESR tubes are available.

Green Top

Green stopper tubes contain the anticoagulant heparin combined with sodium, lithium, or ammonium ion. Heparin prevents clotting by inhibiting thrombin in the coagulation cascade **(see Fig. 2-6).** Tubes should be mixed eight times by gentle inversion to mix the sample and to prevent hemolysis. Green stopper tubes are used for chemistry tests performed on whole blood or plasma. Interference by sodium and lithium heparin with their corresponding chemical tests and by ammonium heparin in blood urea nitrogen (BUN) determinations must be avoided. Green stopper tubes are not used for hematology because heparin interferes with the Wright stained blood smear used for differentials.

Green PST

Light green stopper tubes (BD) contain lithium heparin and a separation gel and are called **plasma separator tubes** (PST). PST tubes are used for plasma determinations in chemistry. They are well suited for potassium determinations because heparin prevents the release of potassium by platelets during clotting and the gel prevents contamination of the plasma by red blood cell potassium. Mix by gentle inversion eight times. The Greiner Bio-One VACUETTE heparin gel tubes have green plastic stoppers with a yellow ring.

TECHNICAL TIP 2-12

Tubes containing a gel barrier may be referred to as PST or SST tubes or as gel barrier tubes, depending on the manufacturer.

Gray Top

Gray stopper tubes are available with a variety of additives and anticoagulants for the primary purpose of preserving glucose. All gray stopper tubes contain a glucose preservative **(antiglycolytic agent),** sodium fluoride. Sodium fluoride maintains glucose for 24 hours. Sodium fluoride is not an anticoagulant; therefore, if plasma is needed for analysis, anticoagulant must also be present. In gray stopper tubes, the anticoagulant is potassium oxalate or Na_2EDTA that prevents clotting by binding calcium. Gray stopper tubes with only sodium fluoride for serum testing are available. When monitoring patient glucose levels, tubes for the collection of plasma and serum should not be interchanged. Gray stopper tubes should not be used for other chemical analyses because sodium fluoride interferes with some enzyme analyses that include creatine kinase (CK), alanine aminotransferase (ALT), aspartate aminotransferase (AST), or alkaline phosphatase (ALP). Gray stopper tubes are not used in hematology because potassium oxalate distorts cellular morphology.

Blood alcohol levels are drawn in gray stopper tubes containing sodium fluoride because microbial growth, which could produce alcohol as a metabolic end product, is inhibited. Tubes with or without potassium oxalate can be used, depending on the need for plasma or serum in the test procedure. Tubes are mixed eight times by gentle inversion.

Royal Blue Top

Royal blue stopper tubes are used for trace elements, toxicology, and nutrient determinations. Because many of the elements analyzed in these studies are significant at very low levels, the tubes must be chemically clean to prevent contamination from the stopper material that could falsely elevate test results. The rubber stoppers are specially formulated to contain the lowest possible levels of metal or other contaminants. Royal blue stopper tubes are available with a spray-coated silica clot activator for serum, or with sodium heparin (Greiner Bio-One VACUETTE) or K_2EDTA (BD) for plasma to conform to a variety of testing requirements. Tube labels are color-coded to indicate the type of additive or anticoagulant in the tube. Invert tubes with anticoagulants eight times and tubes with a clot activator five times to mix.

Tan Top

Tan stopper tubes are available for lead determinations. They are certified to contain less than 0.01 mcg/mL (parts per million [ppm]) lead. The tubes contain K_2EDTA anticoagulant and must be inverted eight times for proper mixing.

Yellow Top

Yellow stopper tubes are available for two different purposes and contain different additives. Yellow stoppers tubes containing the red blood cell preservative acid citrate dextrose (ACD) are used for blood bank special cellular studies, human leukocyte antigen (HLA) phenotyping, and DNA and paternity testing. The acid citrate prevents clotting by binding calcium and the dextrose preserves the red blood cells. The tubes should be inverted eight times.

Sterile **yellow** stopper tubes containing the anticoagulant sodium polyanethol sulfonate (SPS) are used to collect samples to be cultured for the presence of microorganisms. SPS aids in the recovery of microorganisms by inhibiting the actions of complement, phagocytes, and certain antibiotics. SPS also binds calcium to prevent coagulation **(see Fig. 2-6)**. The tube should be inverted eight times.

Light Blue/Black Top

Light blue/black stopper glass tubes contain the anticoagulant sodium citrate, a polyester gel, and a density gradient liquid and are cell preparation tubes (CPT). CPTs are specialty single tube systems used for whole blood molecular diagnostics testing so that mononuclear cells can be separated from whole blood and transported without removing them from the tube. The mononuclear cells and platelets are separated from the granulocytes and red blood cells by the polyester gel and dense gradient liquid when centrifuged. The tube should be inverted eight times.

Red/Green Top

Red/green stopper glass tubes contain the anticoagulant sodium heparin, a polyester gel, and density gradient liquid and are also CPTs. This tube is used for whole blood molecular diagnostic testing when the testing methodology requires heparinized blood. The tube is mixed by inverting eight times.

Orange Top

Orange stoppers are found on tubes containing the clot activator thrombin. The addition of thrombin to the tube results in faster clot formation, usually within 5 minutes. Tubes containing thrombin are used for STAT serum chemistry determinations and on samples from patients receiving anticoagulant therapy. Tubes should be inverted eight times.

Orange stopper tubes containing a thrombin and a separation gel are called rapid serum tubes (RSTs). RSTs tubes clot within 5 minutes and are centrifuged for 10 minutes at a high speed, yielding serum in a short period of time, which is ideal for STAT serum chemistry testing. Tubes should be inverted five times.

Serum Separator Tubes (Gold, Red/gray, Red)

Red/gray and gold stoppers (BD) are found on tubes containing a clot activator and a polymer separation gel. They are referred to as **serum separator tubes (SST).** The tubes contain silica that increases platelet activation, thereby shortening the time required for clot formation. Tubes should be inverted five times to expose the blood to the clot activator. A barrier polymer gel that undergoes a temporary change in viscosity during centrifugation is located at the bottom of the tube. As shown in **Figure 2-29,** when the tube is centrifuged, the gel forms a barrier between the cells and serum to prevent contamination of the serum with cellular materials. To produce a solid separation barrier, samples must be allowed to clot completely before centrifuging. Blood-clotting time is usually 30 minutes and samples should be centrifuged as soon as clot formation is complete. SST tubes are used for chemistry tests. They prevent contamination of the serum by cellular chemicals and products of cellular metabolism. They are not suitable for blood bank and certain immunology/serology tests. The Greiner Bio-One VACUETTE serum gel tubes have red plastic stoppers with yellow rings.

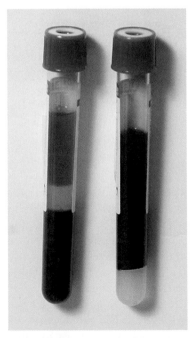

FIGURE 2-29 VACUETTE serum gel tubes before and after collection and centrifugation. *(Reproduced with permission from Strasinger, S.K., and Di Lorenzo, M.S.: The Phlebotomy Textbook, ed. 3. Philadelphia, F.A. Davis, 2011.)*

Red Top

Red stopper plastic tubes contain silica as a clot activator. They are used for serum chemistry tests, serology tests, and in blood banks, where both serum and red blood cells may be used where the gel from the SST tube may interfere. The tubes are inverted five times to initiate the clotting process.

Red stopper glass tubes are often referred to as clot or plain tubes because they contain no anticoagulants or additives. Blood collected in red stopper glass tubes clots by the normal coagulation process in about 60 minutes. Centrifugation of the sample then yields serum as the liquid portion. Red stopper tubes are used for the same purpose as the red plastic tubes. There is no need to invert glass red stopper tubes.

Red/light Gray Top

Red/light gray stopper tubes with clear Hemogard closures are plain tubes because they contain no anticoagulants, additives, or gel. They are used as a discard tube for priming winged blood collection sets for coagulation tests or secondary sample collection tube **(Figs. 2-30 and 2-31).** No inverting of the tube is required.

Evacuated tubes are summarized in **Table 2-1.** Appendix A lists laboratory tests and the required types of anticoagulants and volume of blood required.

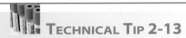

TECHNICAL TIP 2-13

Centrifugation of an incompletely clotted SST tube can produce a nonintact gel barrier and possible cellular contamination of the serum.

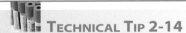

TECHNICAL TIP 2-14

Serum tubes with clot activator cannot be used as a discard tube for coagulation studies.

ORDER OF DRAW

Often several tests are ordered on patients, and blood must be collected in different tubes. The order in which tubes are drawn is one of the most important considerations when collecting blood samples, as this can affect

Hemogard™ Closure	Conventional Stopper	Additive	Inv*	Laboratory Use	Notes
Gold	Red/ Gray	• Clot activator and gel for serum separation	5	For serum determinations in chemistry. Blood clotting time: 30 minutes.	
Light Green	Green/ Gray	• Lithium heparin and gel for plasma separation	8	For plasma determinations in chemistry.	
Red	Red	• Silicone coated (glass) • Clot activator, silicone coated (plastic)	0 5	For serum determinations in chemistry. Blood clotting time, glass: 60 minutes. Blood clotting time, plastic: 30 minutes.	
Orange		• Thrombin-based clot activator with gel for serum separation	5 to 6	For stat serum determinations in chemistry. Blood clotting time: 5 minutes.	
Orange		• Thrombin-based clot activator	8	For stat serum determinations in chemistry. Blood clotting time: 5 minutes.	
Royal Blue		• Clot activator (plastic serum) • K_2EDTA (plastic)	5 8	For trace-element, toxicology, and nutritional-chemistry determinations.	
Green	Green	• Sodium heparin • Lithium heparin	8 8	For plasma determinations in chemistry.	
Gray	Gray	• Potassium oxalate/ sodium fluoride • Sodium fluoride/ Na_2 EDTA • Sodium fluoride (serum tube)	8 8 8	For glucose determinations.	
Tan		• K_2EDTA (plastic)	8	For lead determinations.	
Lavender	Lavender	• Liquid K_3EDTA (glass) • Spray-coated K_2EDTA (plastic)	8 8	For whole blood hematology determinations.	
	Yellow	• Sodium polyanethol sulfonate (SPS) • Acid citrate dextrose additives (ACD): **Solution A** 22.0 g/L trisodium citrate, 8.0 g/L citric acid, 24.5 g/L dextrose **Solution B** 13.2 g/L trisodium citrate, 4.8 g/L citric acid, 14.7 g/L dextrose	8 8 8	SPS for blood culture specimens in microbiology. ACD for blood bank studies, HLA phenotyping, and DNA and paternity testing.	
White		• K_2EDTA and gel for plasma separation	8	For use in molecular diagnostic test methods.	
Pink	Pink	• Spray-coated K_2EDTA (plastic)	8	For whole blood immunohematology testing. Special cross-match label.	
Light Blue / Clear	Light Blue / Light Blue	• Buffered sodium citrate 0.105 M (3.2%) glass 0.109 M (3.2%) plastic • Citrate, theophylline, adenosine, dipyridamole (CTAD)	3–4 3–4	For coagulation determinations.	
Clear	Red/ Light Gray	• None (plastic)	0	For use as a discard tube or secondary specimen tube.	

FIGURE 2-30 BD Vacutainer Venous Blood Collection Tube Guide. *(Reproduced with permission from Strasinger, S.K., and Di Lorenzo, M.S.: Phlebotomy Notes: Pocket Guide to Blood Collection. Philadelphia, FA Davis, 2013.)*

*Inversions at blood collection

Cap Color	Additive	Number of Inversions	Testing Disciplines	Comments
	No additive	5–10	Discard tube Transport/Storage Immunohematology Viral Markers	
	Sodium Citrate 3.2% (0.109 M) 3.8% (0.129 M)	4	Coagulation	If a winged blood collection set is used AND the coagulation specimen is drawn first, a discard tube is recommended to be drawn prior to this tube to ensure the proper anticoagulant-to-blood ratio.*
	Clot Activator	5–10	Chemistry Immunochemistry Immunohematology Viral Markers	For complete clotting, 30 minutes minimum clotting time is required. Incomplete or delayed mixing may result in delayed clotting.
	Clot Activator w/Gel	5–10	Chemistry Immunochemistry TDMs	For complete clotting, 30 minutes minimum clotting time is required. Incomplete or delayed mixing may result in delayed clotting.
	Lithium Heparin Lithium Heparin w/Gel Sodium Heparin	5–10	Chemistry Immunochemistry	
	K_3EDTA K_2EDTA	8–10	Hematology Immunohematology Molecular Diagnostics Viral Markers	
	K_2EDTA gel	8–10	Molecular Diagnostics	
	Sodium Fluoride/ Potassium Oxalate	5–10	Chemisty	
	Sodium Heparin No Additive	5–10	Trace Elements	

Centrifugation Recommendations		
VACUETTE® Serum Tubes (Clot Activator, No Additive)	Min. 1500 g	10 min.
VACUETTE® Serum Clot Activator w/Gel Tubes	1800 g	10 min.
VACUETTE® K_2EDTA w/Gel Tubes	1800 – 2200 g	10 min.
VACUETTE® Plasma Tubes (Lithium or Sodium Heparin, NaF/KO)	2000 - 3000 g	15 min.
VACUETTE® Lithium Heparin w/Gel Tubes	2200 g	15 min.
VACUETTE® Coagulation Tubes (Sodium Citrate)		
Platelet tests (PRP)	150 g	5 min.
Platelet tests (PRP)	1500 - 2000 g	10 min.
Preparation for deep freeze plasma (PFP)	2500 - 3000 g	20 min.

Ring Indicator ● yellow Gel Separation ● black Standard Draw ◉ white Pediatric Draw (2 mL or less)

*CLSI H3-A6 Procedures for the Collection of Diagnostic Blood Specimens by Venipuncture; Approved Standard – 6th Edition

FIGURE 2-31 VACUETTE Tube Guide. *(From Strasinger, S.K., and Di Lorenzo, M.S.: Phlebotomy Notes: Pocket Guide to Blood Collection. Philadelphia, FA Davis, 2013. Courtesy and © Grenier Bio-One. Adapted with permission.)*

TABLE 2-1 Summary of Evacuated Tubes

Stopper Color	Anticoagulant/Additive	Sample Type	Laboratory Use
Lavender	Ethylenediaminetetraacetic acid (EDTA)	Whole blood/plasma	Hematology
Pink	EDTA	Whole blood/plasma	Blood bank
White	EDTA and gel	Plasma	Molecular diagnostics
Light blue	Sodium citrate	Plasma	Coagulation
Red/gray, gold stopper	Clot activator and gel	Serum	Chemistry

TABLE 2-1 Summary of Evacuated Tubes—cont'd

Stopper Color	Anticoagulant/Additive	Sample Type	Laboratory Use
Green	Ammonium heparin	Whole blood/plasma	Chemistry
	Lithium heparin	Whole blood/plasma	
	Sodium heparin	Whole blood/plasma	
Light green	Lithium heparin and gel	Plasma	Chemistry
Red (glass)	None	Serum	Blood bank, chemistry, serology
Red (plastic)	Clot activator	Serum	Blood bank, chemistry, serology
Orange	Thrombin and gel	Serum	Chemistry
Gray	Potassium oxalate/sodium fluoride	Plasma	Chemistry glucose tests, alcohol
	Sodium fluoride	Serum	
	Sodium fluoride/Na_2EDTA	Plasma	
Tan	K_2EDTA	Plasma	Chemistry lead tests
Royal blue	Sodium heparin	Plasma	Chemistry trace elements, toxicology, and nutrient analyses
	K_2EDTA	Plasma	
	Clot activator	Serum	
Yellow	Sodium polyanethol sulfonate (SPS)	Whole blood	Microbiology blood cultures
	Acid citrate dextrose (ACD)	Whole blood	Blood bank
Black	Sodium citrate	Whole blood	Hematology sedimentation rates
Red/light gray/clear	None		Discard tube

some test results **(Fig. 2-32).** Tubes must be collected in a specific order to prevent invalid test results caused by contamination of the sample by microorganisms, tissue thromboplastin, or carryover of additives or anticoagulants between tubes.

For example, the release of tissue thromboplastin from the skin as it is punctured can result in its presence in the first tube collected, and this could interfere with coagulation tests. For some coagulation studies, a discard tube must be drawn before a light blue stopper tube. However, recent studies suggest that the discard tube may no longer be necessary for routine coagulation tests (activated partial thromboplastin time [APTT] and prothrombin time [PT]) unless the draw is difficult or when using a winged blood collection set, but it is still required for special coagulation tests. It is important that the blood collector follow the blood collection protocol of the facility.

Transfer of anticoagulants when changing tubes as a result of possible contamination of the stopper-puncturing needle must be avoided. Blood remaining on the needle

after puncturing a tube can be transferred to the next tube. This is why the discard tube is drawn before the coagulation tube and why tubes containing anticoagulants are drawn after the light blue stopper tube. When one considers the mechanisms of anticoagulation and the chemical composition of the various anticoagulants, it can be understood that the results of several frequently requested tests could be compromised by contamination. For example, contamination of a green, red, or gold stopper tube designated for sodium, potassium, and calcium determinations with EDTA, sodium citrate, or potassium oxalate would falsely decrease the calcium and elevate the sodium or potassium results. Holding blood collection tubes in a downward position to ensure that the tubes fill from the bottom up helps avoid the transfer of anticoagulants from tube to tube. **Box 2-2** lists tests potentially affected by anticoagulant or additive contamination.

When sterile samples, such as blood cultures, are to be collected, they must be considered in the order of draw. Such samples are always drawn first in a sterile

Order	Tube Color	Additive
1	Yellow	SPS Sterile media bottles
2	Light blue	Sodium citrate
3	Red plastic	Clot activator
	Red glass	No additive
	Red and gray SST	Gel separator tube with clot activator
	Gold SST	Gel separator tube with clot activator
	Orange RST	Gel separator tube with thrombin
	Royal blue	Clot activator
4	Light green PST	Gel separator tube with heparin
	Green	Heparin
	Royal blue	Heparin
5	Lavender	EDTA
	Pink	EDTA
	Tan	EDTA
	Royal blue	EDTA
	White PPT	Gel separator with EDTA
6	Gray	Potassium oxalate Sodium fluoride
7	Yellow	ACD

FIGURE 2-32 CLSI Recommended Order of Draw. *(Reproduced with permission from Strasinger, S.K., and Di Lorenzo, M.S.: Phlebotomy Notes: Pocket Guide to Blood Collection. Philadelphia, FA Davis, 2013.)*

bottle or tube to prevent microbial contamination of the stopper-puncturing needle from the unsterile stoppers of tubes used for the collection of other tests.

The CLSI recommends the following order of draw for both ETS and when filling tubes from a syringe:

- Sterile samples (yellow [SPS], blood culture bottles)
- Light blue stopper tubes (sodium citrate)
- Serum tubes: Red/gray SST, gold SST, red plastic stopper tubes (clot activator), and red stopper glass tubes, orange RST (thrombin clot activator with gel), royal blue stopper tubes with clot activator
- Green stopper tubes and light green PST tubes (heparin), royal blue stopper tubes with heparin
- Lavender, pink, white (PPT), tan, and royal blue stopper tubes (EDTA)
- Gray stopper tubes (oxalate, fluoride)
- Yellow stopper tubes (ACD)

SYRINGES

Syringes may be preferred over an ETS when drawing blood from patients with small or fragile veins. The advantage of this system is that the amount of suction pressure on the vein can be controlled by slowly pulling back the syringe plunger.

BOX 2-2 Tests Affected by Anticoagulant/Additive Contamination

EDTA

Alkaline phosphatase (ALP)
Calcium
Activated partial thromboplastin time (APTT)
Creatine kinase-MB (CK-MB)
Potassium
Prothrombin time
Iron
Iron-binding capacity
Sodium
Amylase
Alpha-1-antitrypsin
Cholinesterase
Ceruloplasmin
Uric acid
Creatinine
Copper
Lipase
Lipids
Acid phosphatase

HEPARIN

Activated clotting time
Activated partial thromboplastin time (APTT)
Acid phosphatase
Erythrocyte sedimentation rate (ESR)
Prothrombin time (PT)
Sodium (sodium heparin)
Lithium (lithium heparin)
Blood urea nitrogen (BUN) (ammonium heparin)
Ammonia (ammonium heparin)
Albumin
Cholinesterase
CK-MB
Iron
Gamma-glutamyl transferase (gamma-GT)

POTASSIUM OXALATE

Potassium
Red blood cell morphology
Acid phosphatase

BOX 2-2 Tests Affected by Anticoagulant/Additive Contamination—cont'd

Amylase
Calcium
Lactate dehydrogenase (LD)
Prothrombin time (PT)
Activated partial thromboplastin time (APTT)
Alkaline phosphatase (ALP)
Bilirubin
Creatine kinase (CK)
CK-MB
Insulin
Copper
Low-density lipoprotein (LDL) cholesterol
Lipid electrophoresis
Lithium
Sodium
Protein electrophoresis
T_3 (triiodothyronine)
Triglycerides
Vitamin B_{12}
Iron
Gamma-GT

Sodium Citrate

Alkaline phosphatase (ALP)
Calcium
Phosphorus
Amylase
Alpha-1-antitrypsin
Bilirubin
Cholesterol
Creatine kinase (CK)
CK-MB
Iron
Gamma-GT
Glucose

Uric acid
High-density lipoprotein (HDL) cholesterol
Creatinine
Copper
Sodium
Acid phosphatase
Triglycerides

Sodium Fluoride

Alanine aminotransferase (ALT)
Aspartate aminotransferase (AST)
BUN
Bilirubin
Sodium
Alkaline phosphatase (ALP)
Amylase
Cholesterol
Cholinesterase
Creatine kinase (CK)
CK-MB
Gamma-GT
Uric acid
HDL cholesterol
Creatinine
Copper
Lactate dehydrogenase (LD)
Acid phosphatase
Triglycerides

Clot Activator (Silica)

Activated partial thromboplastin time (APTT)
Prothrombin time (PT)

Reproduced with permission from Strasinger, S.K., and Di Lorenzo, M.S.: The Phlebotomy Textbook, ed. 3. Philadelphia, F.A. Davis, 2011.

Syringes consist of a barrel graduated in milliliters (mL) and a plunger that fits tightly within the barrel creating a vacuum when retracted **(Fig. 2-33).** Syringes used for venipuncture range from 2 to 10 mL, and the blood collector should use a size that corresponds to the amount of blood needed. Needles are attached to a plastic hub designed to fit on the barrel of the syringe. The technique for use of syringes is discussed in Chapter 3.

Syringes that provide a protective sheath to cover the needle before disposal are available. Examples of

safety devices for syringe needles include the Hypodermic Needle-Pro (Smiths Medical, St. Paul, MN), the BD Hypodermic Eclipse needle, and the BD SafetyGlide hypodermic needle (Becton, Dickinson, Franklin Lakes, NJ).

Blood drawn in a syringe must be immediately transferred to appropriate evacuated tubes to prevent the formation of clots. According to the CLSI standards, it is not acceptable to puncture the rubber stopper of the collection tube with the syringe needle and allow the blood

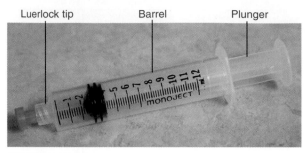

Luerlock tip   Barrel   Plunger

FIGURE 2-33 Diagram of a syringe. *(Reproduced with permission from Strasinger, S.K., and Di Lorenzo, M.S.: The Phlebotomy Textbook, ed. 3. Philadelphia, F.A. Davis, 2011.)*

to be drawn into the tube. A blood transfer device provides a safe means for blood transfer without using the syringe needle or removing the tube stopper. It is an evacuated tube holder with a rubber-sheathed needle inside **(Fig. 2-34)**. After blood collection, the syringe tip is inserted into the hub of the device and evacuated tubes are filled by pushing them on to the rubber-sheathed needle in the holder as in an ETS **(Fig. 2-35)**. The entire syringe/holder assembly is discarded in the sharps container after use. Only syringes with built-in needle protection devices should be used with this system. The safety device must be activated immediately when the needle is removed from the vein to avoid accidental needlesticks. When tubes are filled from a syringe, the CLSI recommends that tubes be filled in the same order as recommended for the order of draw previously listed.

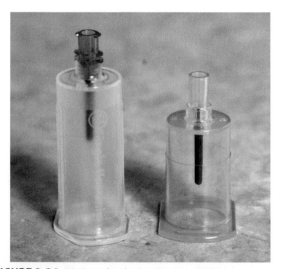

FIGURE 2-34 BD Transfer device (Becton, Dickinson, Franklin Lakes, NJ) and Saf-T Holder device (Smiths Medical, St. Paul, MN). *(Reproduced with permission from Strasinger, S.K., and Di Lorenzo, M.S.: The Phlebotomy Textbook, ed. 3. Philadelphia, F.A. Davis, 2011.)*

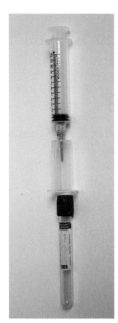

FIGURE 2-35 BD blood transfer device with syringe and evacuated tube. *(Reproduced with permission from Strasinger, S.K., and Di Lorenzo, M.S.: The Phlebotomy Textbook, ed. 3. Philadelphia, F.A. Davis, 2011.)*

 TECHNICAL TIP 2-15

Let the vacuum in the evacuated tube draw the appropriate amount of blood into the tube. Discard any extra blood left in the syringe; do not force it into the tube.

 SAFETY TIP 2-8

Do not unthread the syringe from the blood transfer device. Place the entire assembly in a sharps container. Use a safety needle device with this system.

WINGED BLOOD COLLECTION SETS

Winged blood collection sets, or butterflies as they are routinely called, are used for the following:

- Infusing IV fluids
- Performing venipuncture from very small veins
- Obtaining samples from children and the elderly

Winged blood collection needles used for phlebotomy are usually 23-gauge with lengths of 1/2 to 3/4 of an inch. Plastic attachments to the needle, which resemble "butterfly wings," are used for holding the needle during insertion and to secure the apparatus during use. They also provide the ability to lower the needle insertion angle when working with very small veins. To accommodate the dual purpose of venipuncture and infusion, the needle is attached to flexible plastic tubing that can be attached to an IV setup, syringe, or specially designed evacuated tube holders **(Fig. 2-36).**

There are several winged blood collection needle sets with safety devices built into the system **(Fig. 2-37).** The Vacutainer Safety-Lok (Becton, Dickinson) uses a translucent protective shield that covers the needle immediately after removal from the vein. After use, the needle is completely retracted into the protective shield and locked in place by pushing the yellow shield forward. The BD Vacutainer Push Button Collection Set uses in-vein activation of the needle. The needle is automatically retracted into the device when the blood collector pushes the activation button with the index finger while the needle is still in the vein. The Greiner Bio-One VACUETTE Safety Blood Collection Set is activated by depressing both sides of the stopper and sliding it until

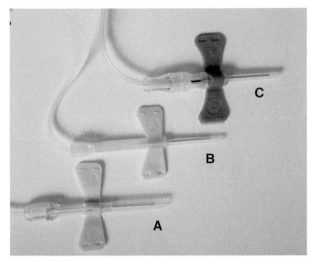

FIGURE 2-37 Examples of winged blood collection needs. *A,* VACUETTE Safety Blood Collection Set (Greiner Bio-One, Kremsmuster, Austria). *B,* BD Vacutainer Safety-Lok Blood Collection Set (Becton, Dickinson, Franklin Lakes, NJ). *C,* BD Vacutainer Push Button Blood Collection Set (Becton, Dickinson, Franklin Lakes, NJ).

the tip of the needle is retracted and covered by the protective shield. Another needle set is the Monoject Angel Wing Blood Collection Set (Kendall, Mansfield, MA). When the needle is withdrawn, a stainless steel safety shield is activated and locks in place to cover the needle. The Puncture Guard winged blood collection set (Gaven Medical, Vernon, CT) produces a safety device that blunts the needle before withdrawal from the vein.

The technique for the use of winged blood collection sets is covered in Chapter 3.

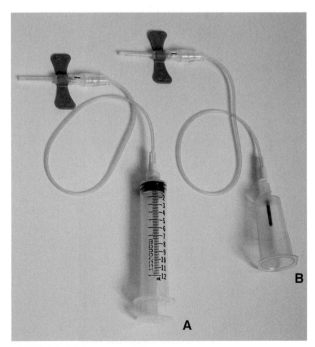

FIGURE 2-36 Winged blood collection sets. *A,* **Attached to a syringe.** *B,* **Attached to an evacuated tube holder.** *(Reproduced with permission from Strasinger, S.K., and Di Lorenzo, M.S.: The Phlebotomy Textbook, ed. 3. Philadelphia, F.A. Davis, 2011.)*

 SAFETY TIP 2-9

Extreme care must be taken when working with winged blood collection sets to avoid accidental needle punctures. Always hold the apparatus by the needle wings and not by the tubing.

 TECHNICAL TIP 2-16

A clear "discard" tube should be drawn before tubes that are affected by an incorrect blood-to-anticoagulant ratio. Air in the winged blood collection set tubing will cause the first tube collected to underfill.

TECHNICAL TIP 2-17

When using a winged blood collection set for blood cultures, the aerobic bottle must be filled first because the addition of air from the tubing will kill any anaerobic organisms present.

TOURNIQUETS

Tourniquets are used during venipuncture to make it easier to locate a patient's veins. They do this by impeding venous, but not arterial, blood flow in the area just below the tourniquet application site. The distended vein then becomes more visible and palpable. Tourniquets are available in various sizes.

The most frequently used tourniquets are one-time use flat nonlatex strips **(Fig. 2-38).** Latex-free tourniquets are available on a roll that is perforated. The stretch tourniquet is used and discarded. Blood pressure cuffs also can be used as tourniquets. The cuff should be inflated to a pressure of 40 mm Hg to allow blood to flow into but not out of the affected veins. The application of tourniquets and the effects on blood tests are discussed in Chapters 3 and 4.

VEIN-LOCATING DEVICES

Portable devices are available to locate veins that are not easily visible. They are particularly advantageous for the neonatal, pediatric, and frail adult patient populations to avoid multiple needlestick attempts for blood collection and for IV insertion. The Venoscope II **(Fig. 2-39)** and Neonatal Transilluminator (Venoscope, LLC, Lafayette, LA) and the Transillumination Vein Locator (VL-U) (Promedic, McCordsville, IN) use a high-intensity light-emitting diode (LED) light that shines through the patient's subcutaneous tissue to highlight the veins that absorb the light rather than reflect it. The vein stands out as a dark line, allowing the blood collector to note the direction of the vein.

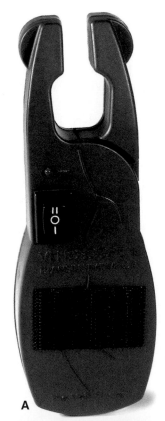

A

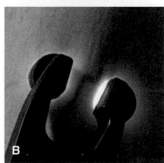

B

FIGURE 2-39 *A,* **Venoscope II transilluminator device.** *B, A* **vein appears as a dark line between the light-emitting arms of the Venoscope.** *(Both courtesy of Venoscope, LLC, Lafayette, LA.)*

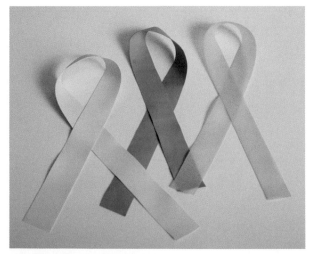

FIGURE 2-38 Various types of tourniquets. *(Reproduced with permission from Strasinger, S.K., and Di Lorenzo, M.S.: The Phlebotomy Textbook, ed. 3. Philadelphia, F.A. Davis, 2011.)*

The blood collector then marks the vein for needle insertion. The Vena-Vue (Biosynergy, Elk Grove Village, IL) uses liquid crystal thermography to locate veins. The device is placed on the skin like a bandage to cool the skin. Heat-emitting veins appear that the blood collector can feel and mark for reassurance. The Vein Entry Indicator Device (VEID) (Vascular Technologies, Ness-Ziona, Israel) uses a sensor technology to indicate correct insertion of a catheter needle in a vein. The device emits a continuous beeping signal, indicating a change of pressure when the needle penetrates a blood vessel. The beeping signal stops when the needle exits the vein.

GLOVES

The Occupational Safety and Health Administration (OSHA) mandates that gloves must be worn when collecting blood and must be changed after each patient. Under routine circumstances, gloves do not need to be sterile. To provide maximal manual dexterity, they should fit securely.

Gloves are available in several varieties. Nonlatex can include nitrile, neoprene, polyethylene, and vinyl **(Fig. 2-40)**. Powdered latex gloves should never be used in blood collection because the glove powder can contaminate some tests and cause latex allergies because the latex particles are suspended in the air when gloves are removed.

ANTISEPTICS

The recommended **antiseptic** used for cleansing the skin in routine blood collection is 70 percent isopropyl alcohol. This is a bacteriostatic antiseptic used to prevent contamination by normal skin bacteria during the short

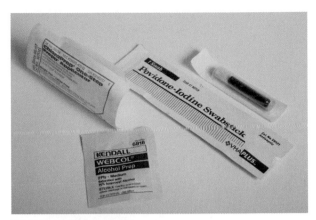

FIGURE 2-41 Antiseptics. *(Reproduced with permission from Strasinger, S.K., and Di Lorenzo, M.S.: The Phlebotomy Textbook, ed. 3. Philadelphia, F.A. Davis, 2011.)*

period required to perform collection of the sample. Individually wrapped prep pads are available for convenience.

Iodine or chlorhexidine gluconate (for patients allergic to iodine) are used to cleanse the site for blood collections that require additional sterility, such as blood cultures **(Fig. 2-41)**. To prevent skin discomfort, iodine should always be removed from the patient's skin with alcohol after a collection procedure.

GAUZE/BANDAGES

Gauze pads that measure 2×2 inches are used for applying pressure to the puncture site immediately after the needle has been removed. Gauze pads also can provide additional pressure when folded in quarters and placed under a bandage. Cotton balls are not recommended because they stick to the site and disrupt the platelet plug when removed, which may reinitiate bleeding. Latex-free bandages or adhesive tape is placed over the puncture site when the bleeding has stopped. Self-adhesive gauze is preferred for patients who are allergic to adhesive bandages, the elderly with thin skin, or when more pressure is required following arterial puncture or blood collection in patients with excessive bleeding. Patients should be instructed to remove the bandage after 15 minutes **(Fig. 2-42)**.

ADDITIONAL SUPPLIES

An essential piece of equipment is a pen for labeling tubes, initialing computer-generated labels, or noting

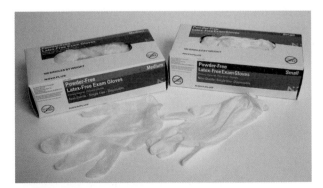

FIGURE 2-40 Gloves. *(Reproduced with permission from Strasinger, S.K., and Di Lorenzo, M.S.: The Phlebotomy Textbook, ed. 3. Philadelphia, F.A. Davis, 2011.)*

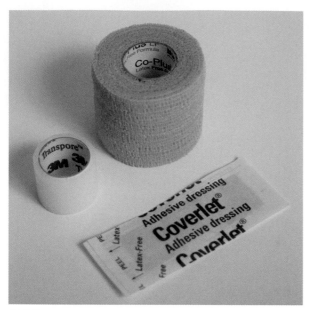

FIGURE 2-42 Bandages. *(Reproduced with permission from Strasinger, S.K., and Di Lorenzo, M.S.: The Phlebotomy Textbook, ed. 3. Philadelphia, F.A. Davis, 2011.)*

unusual circumstances on the requisition form. Biohazard bags should be available for transport of samples based on institutional protocol. Alcohol-based hand sanitizers are an acceptable substitute for hand washing when the hands are not visibly soiled. Wall-mounted hand sanitizers are available in all health-care settings as either gels or foams. Carrying personal bottles of hand sanitizers provides a convenient method of decontamination that is readily available **(Fig. 2-43).**

QUALITY CONTROL

Ensuring the sterility of needles and puncture devices and the stability of evacuated tubes, anticoagulants, and additives is essential to patient safety and sample quality. Disposable needles and puncture devices are individually packaged in tightly sealed sterile containers. Blood collectors should not use puncture equipment if the seal has been broken. Visual inspection for nonpointed or barbed needles may detect manufacturing defects.

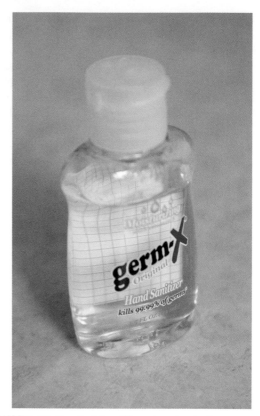

FIGURE 2-43 Handheld sanitizer. *(Reproduced with permission from Strasinger, S.K., and Di Lorenzo, M.S.: The Phlebotomy Textbook, ed. 3. Philadelphia, F.A. Davis, 2011.)*

Manufacturers of evacuated tubes must ensure that tubes, anticoagulants, and additives meet the standards established by the CLSI. Evacuated tubes produced at the same time are referred to as a lot and have a distinguishing lot number printed on the packages. There is also an expiration date printed on each package. The expiration date represents the last day the manufacturer guarantees the stability of the specified amount of vacuum in the tube and the reactivity of the anticoagulants and additives. The expiration date should be checked each time a new package of tubes is opened, and outdated tubes should not be used. Use of expired tubes may cause incompletely filled tubes (short draws), clotted anticoagulated samples, improperly preserved samples, and insecure gel barriers.

 SAFETY TIP 2-10

Blood collectors should not use puncture equipment if the seal has been broken.

 TECHNICAL TIP 2-18

Underfilled EDTA tubes cause red blood cell shrinkage, which will affect hematology tests.

Failure to completely fill tubes (short draws) containing anticoagulants and additives affects sample quality because the amount of anticoagulant or additive present in the tube is based on the assumption that the tube will be completely filled. Possible errors include excessive dilution of the sample by liquid anticoagulants and distortion of cellular structures by increased chemical concentrations.

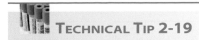

TECHNICAL TIP 2-19

Avoid manual filling of additive tubes to maintain the correct blood-to-anticoagulant ratio.

BIBLIOGRAPHY

Becton, Dickinson Vacutainer Evacuated Blood Collection System. http://www.bd.com

CLSI: *Procedures for the Collection of Diagnostic Blood Specimens by Venipuncture*, ed. 6. Approved Guideline GP41-A6 (H03-A6). Wayne, PA, CLSI, 2007.

CLSI: *Tubes and Additives for Venous and Capillary Blood Specimen Collection*, ed. 6. Approved Standard GP39-A6 (H01-A6). Wayne, PA, CLSI, 2012.

Greiner Bio-One. Venous Blood Collection. http://www.gbo.com

Strasinger, S.K. and DiLorenzo, M.S.: *The Phlebotomy Textbook*, ed. 3. Philadelphia, PA, F.A. Davis Company, 2011.

INTERNET RESOURCES

www.bd.com

www.gavenmedical.com

www.gbo.com

www.kendallhq.com

www.sarstedt.com

www.smiths-medical.com/brands/jelco

www.vacuette.com

www.vanishpoint.com

www.vascula.co.il

www.venoscope.com

VENIPUNCTURE EQUIPMENT SELECTION EXERCISE

INSTRUCTIONS

State or assemble (if requested) the appropriate equipment for the following situations. Include the number and color of evacuated tubes; needle size, syringe size, or winged blood collection set, if appropriate. Instructors may specify the inclusion of supplies. Refer to Appendix A for additional information for this exercise.

1. Collection of a CBC sample from a 35-year-old woman.

   _____

   _____

   _____

2. Collection of a CBC sample from a 3-year-old boy.

   _____

   _____

   _____

3. Collection of samples for a CBC and electrolytes from a 40-year-old man.

   _____

   _____

   _____

4. Collection of a cholesterol sample from the hand of a patient who is taking anticoagulants.

   _____

   _____

   _____

5. Collection of a sample for a coagulation test from an elderly patient.

   _____

   _____

   _____

6. Assemble the equipment to collect a sample for a type and crossmatch on a 50-year-old man.

   _____

   _____

   _____

7. Assemble the equipment to collect a sample for a cardiac risk profile and a prothrombin time from a patient with fragile veins.

   _____

   _____

   _____

8. Assemble the equipment to collect a lead level sample from a 2-year-old patient.

   _____

   _____

   _____

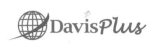 For additional material, please visit http://davisplus.fadavis.com.

REVIEW QUESTIONS

1. The possibility of hemolysis is increased with the use of a:
   a. 16-gauge needle
   b. 21-gauge needle
   c. 23-gauge needle
   d. 25-gauge needle

2. Pushing an evacuated tube through the stopper tube puncturing needle before entering the vein will result in:
   a. Collection of a hemolyzed sample
   b. Quicker collection of the sample
   c. Inability to engage the safety device
   d. Failure to obtain the sample

3. Upon completion of the blood collection, the holder is:
   a. Disinfected with hypochlorite
   b. Discarded in a different container than the needle is discarded in
   c. Discarded with the needle attached
   d. Returned to the collection tray

4. Failure to gently and immediately mix an anticoagulated sample will result in:
   a. Hemolysis
   b. Clot formation
   c. Loss of sterility
   d. Elevated test results

5. Which of the following tubes will automatically be rejected by the laboratory if it is not completely filled?
   a. Light blue
   b. Gray
   c. Red/gray
   d. Light green

6. All of the following tubes contain separation gel except:
   a. Gold stopper tubes
   b. Light green stopper tubes
   c. Lavender stopper tubes
   d. White stopper tubes

7. You receive a requisition for the following tubes: light blue, lavender, green, and red. In what order should the tubes be drawn?
   a. Green, light blue, red, lavender
   b. Light blue, red, green, lavender
   c. Red, green, light blue, lavender
   d. Lavender, red, green, light blue

8. When transferring blood from a syringe to an evacuated tube, the recommended method is to:
   a. Use a blood transfer device
   b. Puncture the tube stopper
   c. Change needles and puncture the stopper
   d. Remove the tube stopper and the needle

9. The recommended antiseptic for routine venipuncture is:
   a. Chlorhexidine gluconate
   b. Isopropyl alcohol
   c. Antimicrobial soap
   d. Iodine

10. Using evacuated tubes past their expiration date may result in:
    a. Hemolyzed samples
    b. Incompletely filled tubes
    c. Secure gel barriers
    d. Overfilled tubes

FOR FURTHER STUDY

1. Can a lavender stopper tube be used to perform a prothrombin time? Why or why not?

2. Why would a chemistry department reject an SST tube into which blood from a syringe has been transferred?

3. Why is an SST tube preferred over a red stopper tube for chemistry tests?

4. What is the name of the fluid obtained when centrifuging a blood collection tube containing an anticoagulant? Does this fluid contain fibrinogen?

CASE STUDY 2-1

Jane, the blood collector at a physician's clinic, was asked to draw blood for a CBC and electrolytes. The patient, Marcia, had very small, fragile veins, so Sue used a syringe with a 25-gauge needle. The blood was sent to the hospital laboratory via a courier. Joan, the medical laboratory scientist, called the physician's office and reported that the potassium results could not be correct and asked that Marcia's blood be redrawn.

1. What tubes should be collected for the CBC and electrolytes?

2. What is the correct order of tube fill with a syringe?

3. Name two reasons that the potassium would be incorrect.

CASE STUDY 2-2

Sarah, the nurse at a busy internal medicine office, was responsible for collecting blood samples for PT (INR) test requests from patients on Coumadin therapy. She preferred using a winged blood collection set with an evacuated tube holder for these collections. Many of her light blue stopper tubes were rejected, causing the patients to have their blood redrawn.

1. What is the most probable reason for the light blue stopper tubes to be rejected?

2. Name a reason that it can happen when using a winged blood collection set.

3. What could Sarah have done differently?

Venipuncture Techniques

LEARNING OBJECTIVES

Upon completion of this chapter, the reader will be able to:

3.1 List the required information on a requisition form.

3.2 Describe correct patient identification and sample labeling procedures.

3.3 Correctly assemble venipuncture equipment and supplies.

3.4 Name and locate the three most frequently used veins for venipuncture, and describe when these sites would be unacceptable.

3.5 Correctly apply a tourniquet and state why the tourniquet can be applied for only 1 minute.

3.6 List methods used to locate veins that are not prominent.

3.7 Describe the different antiseptics used to cleanse the venipuncture site.

3.8 State the steps in a venipuncture procedure, and correctly perform a routine venipuncture using an evacuated tube system (ETS), syringe system, and winged blood collection set.

3.9 Demonstrate safe disposal of contaminated needles and supplies.

3.10 Deliver samples to the laboratory in a timely manner.

Antecubital Fossa Indentation of the midarm opposite the elbow (location of the large veins used in phlebotomy)

Basilic Vein Vein located on the underside of the arm near the elbow bone

Cephalic Vein Vein located on the thumb side of the arm

Hematoma Discoloration of the skin produced by leakage of blood into the tissue

Hemoconcentration Increase in the ratio of formed elements to plasma

Informed Consent Patient's right to know the method and risks before agreeing to treatment

Mastectomy Removal of a breast

Median Cubital Vein Vein located in the center of the antecubital fossa

Palpation Examination by touch

Petechiae Small red spots appearing on the skin

Requisition Form detailing orders for patient testing and identification

Syncope Fainting

INTRODUCTION

The venipuncture technique consists of a series of steps that, when practiced consistently, provide quality samples and cause minimal patient discomfort. Administrative protocols vary among facilities, and, of course, every patient is different; however, many basic rules are the same in all situations. These basic rules must be followed to ensure the safety of the patient and the person performing the procedure and to produce samples that are representative of the patient's condition.

This chapter presents a detailed description of the recommended steps in the venipuncture procedure and possible complications that could occur at each step.

BLOOD COLLECTION PROCEDURE

Examine the Requisition Form

All blood collection procedures begin with the receipt of a test **requisition** form generated by or at the request of a health-care provider. The requisition is essential to provide the blood collector with the information needed to correctly identify the patient, organize the necessary equipment, collect the appropriate samples, and provide legal protection. Blood samples should not be collected without a requisition form, and this form must accompany the samples sent to the laboratory.

The actual format of a requisition form may vary. Patient information may be handwritten or imprinted on color-coded forms with test check-off lists for different departments **(Fig. 3-1).** There may be multiple copies for purposes of record-keeping and billing. Computer-generated forms may include not only the patient information and tests requested but also the tube labels and bar codes for sample processing, the number and type of collection tubes needed, and any special collection instructions **(Fig. 3-2). Figure 3-3** shows an example of computer-generated labels.

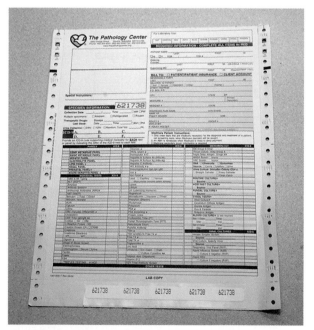

FIGURE 3-1 Manual requisition form. *(Reproduced with permission from Strasinger, S.K., and Di Lorenzo, M.S.: The Phlebotomy Textbook, ed. 3. Philadelphia, F.A. Davis, 2011.)*

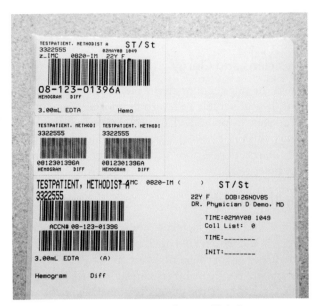

FIGURE 3-2 Sample requisition form and labels. *(Reproduced with permission from Strasinger, S.K., and Di Lorenzo, M.S.: The Phlebotomy Textbook, ed. 3. Philadelphia, F.A. Davis, 2011.)*

FIGURE 3-3 Computer labels printing in the laboratory. *(Reproduced with permission from Strasinger, S.K., and Di Lorenzo, M.S.: The Phlebotomy Textbook, ed. 3. Philadelphia, F.A. Davis, 2011.)*

When working in emergency care, a preprinted requisition form may not be available, making it necessary for the information to be written on a blank form. Be sure to transfer the identification number from the patient's wristband when a temporary identification system has been used. When verbal orders are given, the name of the person giving the order should be documented.

Requisitions must contain certain basic information to ensure that the sample drawn and the test results are correlated to the appropriate patient and the results can be correctly interpreted with regard to any special conditions, such as the time of collection. **Box 3-1** includes required information on a requisition.

TECHNICAL TIP 3-1

Personnel should never collect samples before the generation of a requisition form.

TECHNICAL TIP 3-2

All needed information is provided on labels generated on the computer information system.

Greet the Patient

The blood collector should introduce him- or herself and obtain consent to collect a blood sample. This interaction begins the communication process and develops trust with the patient **(Fig. 3-4).** The procedure must be explained in nontechnical terms and understood by the

---

BOX 3-1 Required Information on a Requisition Form

- Patient's first and last name
- Patient's date of birth
- Patient's identification number
- Patient's accession number
- Patient's location
- Ordering health-care provider's full name
- Tests requested
- Date and time of sample collection
- Special collection information (such as fasting sample or latex sensitivity)
- Special patient information (such as areas that should not be used for venipuncture)
- Number and type of collection tubes
- Status of sample (such as STAT or timed)
- Billing information and ICD-10 codes

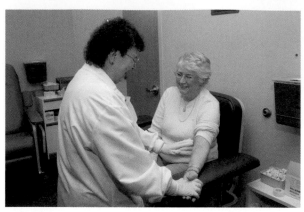

FIGURE 3-4 A blood collector greeting a patient in an outpatient setting. *(Reproduced with permission from Strasinger, S.K., and Di Lorenzo, M.S.: The Phlebotomy Textbook, ed. 3. Philadelphia, F.A. Davis, 2011.)*

patient. The patient expects that the blood collector is competent in blood collection procedures. The patient is then able to give **informed consent** to the procedure. Obtaining consent is as simple as identifying yourself and explaining that you are there to obtain a blood sample from the patient's arm for tests the health-care provider has requested. Consent may be verbal or nonverbal indicated by extending the arm or rolling up the sleeve. According to the Patient Bill of Rights, the patient has the right to refuse. Patient refusal must be documented using the appropriate forms and reported to the patient's nurse. The blood collector may be guilty of assault if the patient perceives that the blood collector is ignoring the refusal.

Sleeping Patients

Whenever possible, patients who are sleeping should be awakened and allowed to orient themselves prior to the procedure. The patient must be awake for accurate identification and to give informed consent for the procedure.

Unconscious Patients

Unconscious patients should be greeted in the same manner as conscious patients, because they may be capable of hearing and understanding even though they cannot respond. In this circumstance, it may be necessary to request assistance from other members of the unit staff, because the patient may move when the needle is inserted.

Psychiatric Units

Psychiatric patients are often anxious about the venipuncture procedure and feel more comfortable when a primary caregiver with whom they are familiar

is present. Be sure to place blood collection equipment away from the patient.

Physicians and Clergy

When the physician or clergy member is with the patient, it is preferable to return at another time, unless the request is for a STAT or timed sample. When this occurs, the blood collector should explain the situation and request permission to perform the procedure at that time.

Family and Visitors

Visitors and family members may be with the patient. They should be greeted in the same manner as the patient and given the option to step outside. However, visitors and family members can sometimes be helpful in the case of pediatric or very apprehensive patients.

Unavailable Patient

If the patient is not in the room, the blood collector should attempt to locate the patient by checking with the nurse. If the sample must be collected at a particular time, it may be possible to draw blood from the patient in the area to which he or she has been taken. If this is not possible, the nurse must be notified and the appropriate forms must be completed so that the test can be rescheduled.

 TECHNICAL TIP 3-3

Good verbal, listening, and nonverbal skills are very important for patient reassurance and trust.

 SAFETY TIP 3-1

A sleeping or unconscious patient may move or jerk unexpectedly when the needle is inserted into the vein or while the needle is in the vein during the venipuncture procedure and cause injury to the patient and the blood collector.

Identify the Patient

The most important step in the venipuncture procedure is the correct identification of the patient. Serious diagnostic or treatment errors and even death can occur when blood is drawn from the wrong patient.

The Clinical and Laboratory Standards Institute (CLSI) recommends two identifiers for patient identification. The College of American Pathologists (CAP) and The Joint Commission (TJC) patient safety goals require a minimum of two identifiers. To ensure that blood is drawn from the right patient, compare the information obtained verbally and from the patient's wrist identification (ID) band with the information on the requisition **(Fig. 3-5).** A wristband lying on the bedside table cannot be used for identification because it could belong to anyone. Likewise, a sign over the patient's bed or on the door cannot be relied on for identification because the patient could be in the wrong bed or room.

TECHNICAL TIP 3-4

Particular attention should be paid to the hospital identification number, because it is possible for two patients to have the same name, date of birth, and health-care provider; however, they could not have the same identification number.

Inpatient Identification

Verbal identification is made after the patient greeting by asking the patient to state his or her first and last name, spell the last name, and give date of birth. Do not ask, "Are you Mr. Jones?" because many patients will say yes to any questions asked. Verify that the computer-generated sample labels match the requisition and patient identification. The CLSI standard GP39-A6 (H3-A6) recommends a third identification check that includes comparing the labeled sample with the patient's identification bracelet or request the patient confirm the tube is properly labeled. This ensures that samples are correctly labeled at the patient's bedside.

For inpatients, examining the information on the patient's wristband, which should be present on all hospitalized patients, follows verbal identification. All information on the wrist ID band must match the information on the requisition form. The information should be identical, and any discrepancies investigated prior to obtaining the sample.

Bar-Code Technology

Positive patient identification can be made using bar-code technology. Using a wireless handheld personal digital assistant (PDA), the blood collector positively identifies the patient by scanning the bar code on the patient's hospital ID band. The patient's identification is matched against a blood collection order on the mobile device, which verifies that a blood sample is required and the correct patient has been identified. The system, which is interfaced with the laboratory information system (LIS), specifies the tests ordered, which kind of tube should be used, and any special handling instructions. After the patient has been properly identified and the blood collected, the patient's hospital ID band is scanned again and the sample label is printed at the bedside. The system detects duplicate draw orders, new test requests, or cancellation of tests. Labels for a specific patient are printed only after the patient has been identified; therefore, the possibility of placing the wrong label on a sample is eliminated.

The newest form of sample identification is radio frequency identification (RFID). RFID tags are small silicon chips that transmit unique patient identification and sample collection information obtained from the LIS to a wireless receiver. RFID tags are attached to the laboratory samples and can be detected at various distances. The system tracks samples as they are being transported to the laboratory.

Missing ID Band

Patients without ID bands attached to their bodies must have the band reapplied prior to sample collection

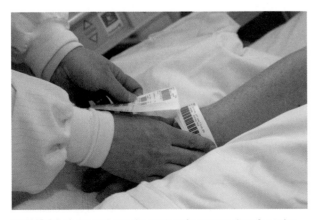

FIGURE 3-5 Identifying the patient by comparing the wrist ID band with the requisition. *(Reproduced with permission from Strasinger, S.K., and Di Lorenzo, M.S.: The Phlebotomy Textbook, ed. 3. Philadelphia, F.A. Davis, 2011.)*

according to the facility's protocol. The name of the person identifying the patient should be documented. In the rare case that a patient cannot wear an ID band or there is not time to place the ID band, the nurse or caregiver must identify the patient and sign the requisition. If a patient is unable to properly identify him- or herself, the CLSI requires a caregiver or family member to provide identification information on the patient's behalf before blood collection. The name of the verifier must be documented. In the cases of drug testing, a photo ID might be required.

Outpatient Identification

In an outpatient setting, comparison of verbal information with the requisition form may be the only means of verifying identification. Ask the patient to state his or her full name, spell the last name, and state his or her address and birth date after calling the patient back to the drawing area. Compare the verbal information with the requisition form to verify the patient's identification. A person who is hard of hearing or nervous about the procedure may stand and follow you to the blood collection area from the waiting room just because you looked at him or her when calling the patient's name even when it was a different person's name that was called. Outpatients traditionally have not worn ID bands; however, facilities are beginning to assign an ID band for outpatient procedures to avoid patient identification errors. Photo identification may be a requirement for certain legal tests. Clinics may provide a patient ID card that can be imprinted or scanned for patient identification and to generate a requisition. Written policies should be available for identifying patients, and these policies must be followed in order to properly perform double identification requirements.

Unidentified Emergency Department Patients

Unidentified patients are sometimes brought into the emergency department (ED), and a system must be in place to ensure they are correctly matched with their laboratory work. The American Association of Blood Banks (AABB) requires that the patient be positively identified with a temporary but clear designation attached to the body. Some hospitals generate ID bands with an ID number and a tentative name, such as John Doe or Patient X. The temporary ID must be placed on all requisitions and samples and must be cross-referenced

with the permanent identification name and number when it becomes available.

Commercial Identification Systems

Commercial identification systems are particularly useful when blood transfusions are required. In these systems, the ID band that is attached to the patient comes with matching identification stickers. The stickers are placed on the sample tubes, the requisition form, and any units of blood designated for the patient. Blood bank identification systems are used in addition to routine ID bands, not instead of them. In some facilities, patients are required to wear the blood bank identification band for 48 hours to indicate how long the sample that has been drawn can be used. Written procedures should be available for using the commercial systems for identifying the patient and sample.

 TECHNICAL TIP 3-5

It is imperative that the information that the blood collector transcribes on the commercial blood bank ID band matches the patient's routine ID band. The blood sample will be rejected if there are any discrepancies.

Identification of Young, Cognitively Impaired, or Patients Who Do Not Speak the Language

If a patient is too young, cognitively impaired, or does not speak the language of the blood collector, ask the patient's nurse, relative, or a friend to identify the patient by name, address, identification number, or date of birth. Document the name of the verifier. This information must be compared with the information on the requisition and the patient's identification band. Any discrepancies must be resolved before collecting the sample.

 SAFETY TIP 3-2

Personnel already familiar with a patient must never become lax with regard to patient identification.

SAFETY TIP 3-3

Long-term care facilities usually do not put identification bands on their residents. Always ask a caregiver or family member to provide the identification information and compare it with the requisition before blood collection.

TECHNICAL TIP 3-6

When necessary, writing down information or using sign language or an interpreter will help the patient to understand the procedure and to give permission for the blood collection.

Prepare the Patient

Reassurance of the patient begins with the greeting and continues throughout the procedure. Provide a brief explanation of the procedure, including any nonroutine techniques that will be used, but do not discuss the actual tests that are to be performed. Patients should not be told that the procedure will be painless.

While talking with the patient, verify that any pretest preparation, such as fasting (nothing to eat or drink except water for 8 to12 hours before the procedure) or abstaining from medications that can interfere with laboratory testing, has occurred. When these procedures have not been followed and the sample is still required after consultation with the nurse or health-care provider, the irregular condition, such as "not fasting," should be noted on the requisition form and on the sample. Ask the patient whether he or she has a latex sensitivity. Use latex-free supplies where appropriate.

Numerous variables associated with a patient's activities prior to sample collection can affect the quality of the sample. The preexamination phase of laboratory testing involves processes that occur before testing of the specimen. Errors that occur during this phase often happen during blood collection and are primarily controlled by the blood collector. These variables can include diet, posture, exercise, stress, alcohol, smoking, time of day, altitude, and medications and are discussed

in Chapter 4. Physiological variables, such as age and gender, also affect reference values for test results. Other patient conditions that may influence laboratory test results are dehydration, fever, and pregnancy. (See Chapter 4.)

Position the Patient

The patient must be positioned conveniently and safely for the procedure. To guard against a possible episode of **syncope,** patients should always be sitting or lying down when phlebotomy is performed.

Outpatients are seated or reclined in a drawing chair as shown in **Figure 3-6,** preferably one with a movable arm that serves the dual purpose of providing a solid surface for the patient's arm and preventing a patient who faints from falling out of the chair. Patients who have had previous difficulties during venipuncture should lie down for the procedure. It is important when collecting a blood sample from a patient in a home setting that the patient be seated in a chair with armrests and the patient's arm placed on a hard surface. A sofa or bed may be used if the patient is anxious or has had previous difficulties during venipuncture.

The arm should be firmly supported and extended downward in a straight line, allowing the tube to fill from the bottom up to prevent reflux and anticoagulant carryover between tubes. Asking the patient to make a fist with the opposite hand and placing it behind the elbow will provide support and make the vein easier to locate. Placing a pillow, towel, or phlebotomy wedge under the patient's arm stabilizes the arm and provides comfortable support **(Fig. 3-7).**

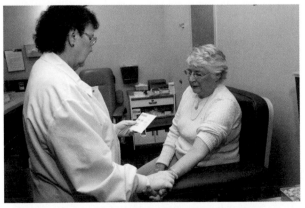

FIGURE 3-6 Patient seated in a blood drawing chair. *(Reproduced with permission from Strasinger, S.K., and Di Lorenzo, M.S.: The Phlebotomy Textbook, ed. 3. Philadelphia, F.A. Davis, 2011.)*

⚠ SAFETY TIP 3-4

Never draw blood from a patient who is in a standing position.

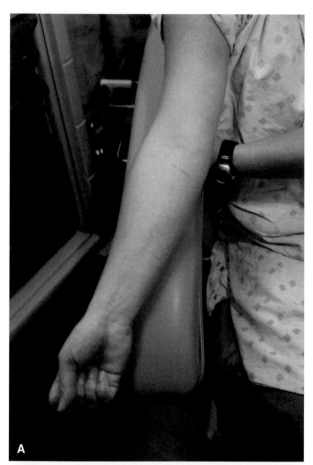

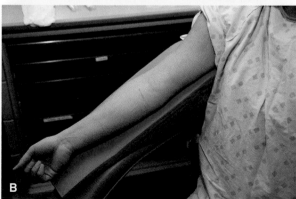

FIGURE 3-7 Positioning the patient's arm. A, Using patient's fist under the arm as a brace. B, Using a phlebotomy wedge.
(Reproduced with permission from Strasinger, S.K., and Di Lorenzo, M.S.: The Phlebotomy Textbook, ed. 3. Philadelphia, F.A. Davis, 2011.)

TECHNICAL TIP 3-7

When supporting the patient's arm, do not hyperextend the elbow. This may make vein palpation difficult. Sometimes bending the elbow very slightly may aid in vein palpation.

Patients should remove any foreign object, such as food, drink, gum, or a thermometer, from his or her mouth before performance of the venipuncture.

Patient Refusal

Some patients may refuse to have their blood drawn, and they have the right to do this. If the patient refuses, this decision should be documented according to the facility policy.

Select Equipment

Before approaching the patient for the actual venipuncture, the blood collector should gather all necessary supplies (including collection equipment, antiseptic pads, gauze pads, bandages, and needle disposal system) and place them close to the patient. The blood collection tray should not be placed on the bed or on the patient's eating table. Place supplies on the same side as your free hand during blood collection to avoid reaching across the patient and causing unnecessary movement of the needle in the patient's vein. Reexamine the requisition form, and select the appropriate number and type of collection tubes. Check the expiration date on each tube and discard any tube that is expired.

Place the tubes in the correct order for sample collection, and have additional tubes readily available for possible use during the procedure **(Fig. 3-8).** It is not uncommon to find an evacuated tube that does not contain the necessary amount of vacuum to collect a full tube of blood. Accidentally pushing a tube past the indicator mark on the holder before the vein is entered also results in loss of vacuum.

Sanitize Hands and Apply Gloves

In front of the patient, the blood collector should sanitize his or her hands and apply clean gloves. Pull gloves over the cuffs of protective clothing (laboratory coat) for maximum protection.

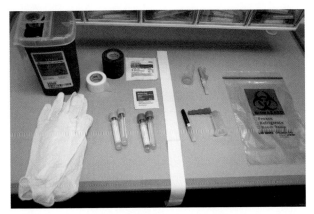

FIGURE 3-8 Venipuncture collection equipment. *(Reproduced with permission from Strasinger, S.K., and Di Lorenzo, M.S.: The Phlebotomy Textbook, ed. 3. Philadelphia, F.A. Davis, 2011.)*

TECHNICAL TIP 3-8

Patients are often reassured that proper safety practices are being followed when gloves are applied in their presence.

SAFETY TIP 3-5

Occupational Safety and Health Administration (OSHA) regulations mandate that gloves be worn when performing a venipuncture procedure.

Apply the Tourniquet

The tourniquet serves two functions in the venipuncture procedure. By causing blood to accumulate in the veins, the tourniquet causes the veins to be more easily located and also provides a larger amount of blood for collection. Use of a tourniquet can alter some test results by increasing the ratio of cellular elements to plasma (**hemoconcentration**) and by causing hemolysis. Therefore, the maximum time a tourniquet should remain in place is 1 minute. This may require that the tourniquet be applied twice during the venipuncture procedure: first when vein selection is being made and then immediately before the puncture is performed. When the tourniquet is used during vein selection, the CLSI recommends that it should be released for 2 minutes before being reapplied.

TECHNICAL TIP 3-9

A tourniquet is used unless it interferes with test results, such as in a lactate test.

Hemoconcentration

Tests most likely to be affected by prolonged tourniquet application are those measuring large molecules, such as plasma proteins and lipids, or analytes affected by hemolysis, including potassium, lactic acid, and enzymes. During multiple tube collections, the tourniquet must be removed when the timing exceeds 1 minute. Tourniquet application and fist clenching are not recommended when drawing samples for lactic acid determinations.

Other causes of hemoconcentration are excessive squeezing or probing a site, long-term IV therapy, sclerosed or occluded veins, and vigorous fist clenching. **Box 3-2** lists the major tests affected by hemoconcentration.

Ideally, the tourniquet should be released as soon as blood begins to flow into the first tube to prevent hemoconcentration and hemolysis. When multiple tubes are collected, the blood collector must make the decision regarding immediately removing the tourniquet based on the size of the patient's veins or the difficulty of the puncture. Regardless of the situation, the tourniquet should not remain in place for longer than 1 minute.

The tourniquet should be placed lying flat on the arm 3 to 4 inches above the venipuncture site. Application of the tourniquet requires practice to develop a smooth technique and can be difficult if properly fitting gloves are not worn. **Procedure 3-1** shows the technique used for strip tourniquet application.

To achieve adequate pressure, both sides of the tourniquet must be grasped near the patient's arm and,

---

BOX 3-2 Tests Affected by Hemoconcentration

Ammonia
Bilirubin
Calcium
Enzymes
Iron
Lactic acid
Lipids
Potassium
Proteins
Red blood cells

while maintaining tension, the left side is tucked under the right side. The loop formed should face downward toward the patient's **antecubital fossa** area, and the free ends of the tourniquet must be pointing away from the venipuncture site to avoid contaminating the site. The tourniquet must be able to be easily released with one hand by pulling the short end forward. Left-handed persons would reverse this procedure.

Tourniquets that are folded or applied too tightly are uncomfortable for the patient and may obstruct blood flow to the area. The appearance of small, reddish discolorations (**petechiae**) on the patient's arm, blanching of the skin around the tourniquet, and the blood collector's inability to feel a radial pulse are indications of a tourniquet tied too tightly.

When dealing with patients with skin conditions or open sores, it may be necessary to place the tourniquet over the patient's gown or to cover the area with gauze or dry cloth prior to application. If possible, another area should be selected for the venipuncture. Do not apply a tourniquet to an arm on the same side as a mastectomy.

A blood pressure cuff is sometimes used to locate veins that are difficult to find. The cuff should be maintained at a pressure of 40 mm Hg.

Technical Tip 3-10

A tourniquet applied too close to the venipuncture site may cause the vein to collapse.

Select the Venipuncture Site

The preferred site for venipuncture is the antecubital fossa located anterior to the elbow. As shown in **Figure 3-9,** the median cubital, cephalic, median cephalic, and basilic veins are located in this area, and, in most patients, at least one of these veins can

---

PROCEDURE 3-1 **Tourniquet Application**

EQUIPMENT:

Vinyl or latex strip tourniquet

PROCEDURE:

Step 1. Position the vinyl or latex strip 3 to 4 inches above the venipuncture site. Avoid areas with a skin lesion or apply the tourniquet over the patient's gown.

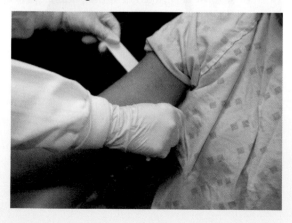

Step 2. Grasp both sides of the tourniquet and, while maintaining tension, cross the tourniquet over the patient's arm.

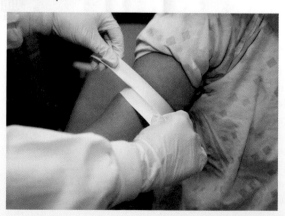

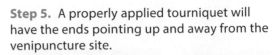

PROCEDURE 3-1 Tourniquet Application (Continued)

Step 3. Hold both ends between the thumb and forefinger of one hand close to the arm.

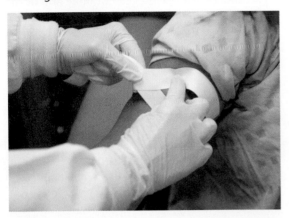

Step 4. Tuck a portion of the left side under the right side to make a partial loop facing the antecubital area.

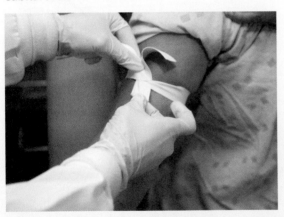

Step 5. A properly applied tourniquet will have the ends pointing up and away from the venipuncture site.

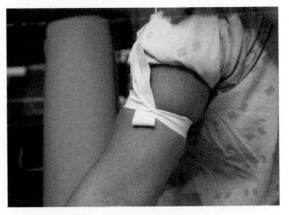

Step 6. Pull the end of the loop to release the tourniquet with one hand. The tourniquet should be on for only 1 minute.

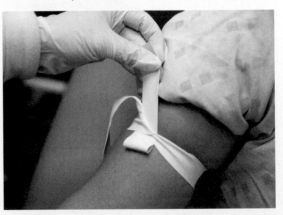

Reproduced with permission from Strasinger, S.K., and Di Lorenzo, M.S.: The Phlebotomy Textbook, ed. 3. Philadelphia, F.A. Davis, 2011.

be easily located. Vein patterns vary among individuals. The most often seen arrangements of veins in the antecubital fossa are referred to as the "H-shaped" and "M-shaped" patterns. The H pattern includes the cephalic, median cubital, and basilic veins in a pattern that looks like a slanted H. The most prominent veins in the M pattern are the cephalic, median cephalic, median basilic, and basilic veins. The H-shaped pattern is seen in approximately 70 percent of the population **(Fig. 3-10)**.

Notice that the veins continue down the forearm to the wrist area; however, in these areas the veins become smaller and less well anchored, and punctures are more painful to the patient. Small, prominent veins are also

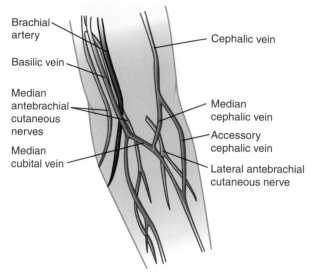

FIGURE 3-9 The veins in the arm most often chosen for venipuncture. *(Reproduced with permission from Strasinger, S.K., and Di Lorenzo, M.S.: The Phlebotomy Textbook, ed. 3. Philadelphia, F.A. Davis, 2011.)*

located in the back of the hand **(Fig. 3-11).** When necessary, these veins can be used for venipuncture but may require a smaller needle or winged blood collection set **(Fig. 3-12).** The veins of the lower arm and hand are also the preferred sites for administering IV fluids because they allow the patient more arm flexibility. Frequent venipuncture in these veins could make them unsuitable for IV use. Some institutions have special ID bands that indicate the restricted use of veins being used for other procedures.

 SAFETY TIP 3-6

The CLSI standards state that veins on the underside of the wrist must not be used for venipuncture, because of the chance of accidentally puncturing arteries, nerves, or tendons.

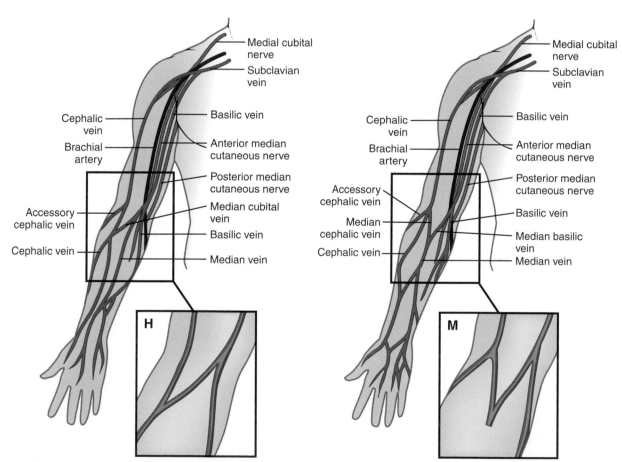

FIGURE 3-10 Major antecubital veins showing the H- and M-shaped patterns. *(Reproduced with permission from Strasinger, S.K., and Di Lorenzo, M.S.: The Phlebotomy Textbook, ed. 3. Philadelphia, F.A. Davis, 2011.)*

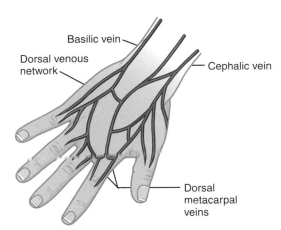

Basilic vein

Dorsal venous network

Cephalic vein

Dorsal metacarpal veins

FIGURE 3-11 Veins on the back of the hand and wrist. *(Reproduced with permission from Strasinger, S.K., and Di Lorenzo, M.S.: The Phlebotomy Textbook, ed. 3. Philadelphia, F.A. Davis, 2011.)*

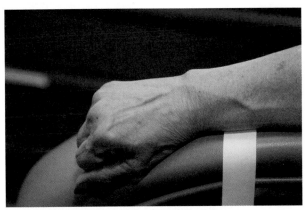

FIGURE 3-12 Prominent hand and wrist veins. *(Reproduced with permission from Strasinger, S.K., and Di Lorenzo, M.S.: The Phlebotomy Textbook, ed. 3. Philadelphia, F.A. Davis, 2011.)*

Median Cubital Vein

Of the veins located in the antecubital fossa, the **median cubital** is the vein of choice because it is large and well anchored, and does not tend to move when the needle is inserted. It is often closer to the surface of the skin, more isolated from underlying structures, and the least painful to puncture because there are fewer nerve endings in this area.

Cephalic Vein

The **cephalic vein,** located on the thumb side of the arm, is usually more difficult to locate, except possibly in larger patients, and has more tendencies to move. The cephalic vein should be the second choice if the median cubital vein is inaccessible in both arms.

 TECHNICAL TIP 3-11

Because the cephalic vein is closer to the surface, there is the possibility of a blood spurt when the needle is inserted into the vein. This often is controlled by decreasing the angle of needle insertion to 15 degrees.

Basilic Vein

The **basilic vein** is located on the inner edge of the antecubital fossa. The basilic vein should be used as the last choice because the median nerve and brachial artery are in close proximity to it, increasing the risk of injury. The basilic vein is the least firmly anchored; therefore, it has a tendency to roll and **hematoma** formation is more likely. The basilic vein is located near the brachial artery, and extreme care must be taken not to accidentally puncture the artery.

 TECHNICAL TIP 3-12

Using a syringe method for blood collection from the basilic vein offers more control over a rolling vein.

 TECHNICAL TIP 3-13

Always locate the brachial pulse before accessing the basilic vein to prevent accidental arterial puncture.

 SAFETY TIP 3-7

Only superficial veins should be used in children.

 SAFETY TIP 3-8

Collecting blood from the basilic vein has caused more complaints, injury, and legal actions to be taken against blood collectors than any other vein.

Two routine steps in the venipuncture procedure aid in locating a suitable vein: applying a tourniquet and asking the patient to make a fist. The tourniquet can be applied for only 1 minute; therefore, after the vein is located, the tourniquet should be removed while the site is being cleansed, and then reapplied immediately before the venipuncture.

TECHNICAL TIP 3-14

Continuous clenching or pumping of the fist is not recommended because it will result in hemoconcentration, altering some test results, such as those for potassium and ionized calcium.

TECHNICAL TIP 3-15

Patients often think they are helping by pumping their fists, because this is an acceptable practice when donating blood. In contrast to laboratory samples, a donated unit of blood is even better when it is hemoconcentrated.

Veins are located by sight and touch, referred to as **palpation.** The ability to feel a vein is much more important than the ability to see a vein. Palpation is performed by using the tip of the index finger of the nondominant hand to probe the antecubital area with a pushing motion rather than a stroking motion. Feel for the vein in both a vertical and horizontal direction.

⚠ SAFETY TIP 3-9

Gloves should be worn when palpating veins to prevent contact with microorganisms, such as methicillin-resistant *Staphylococcus aureus* (MRSA) and vancomycin-resistant enterococci (VRE).

Palpation is used to determine the size, depth, and direction of the vein to aid in directing the needle during insertion. The pressure applied by palpating locates deep veins and distinguishes veins, which feel like spongy, resilient, tubelike structures, from rigid tendon cords. Veins

must be differentiated from arteries, which produce a pulse; therefore, the thumb should not be used to palpate because it has a pulse beat. Turning the arm slightly helps distinguish veins from other structures. Select a vein that is easily palpated and large enough to support good blood flow **(Fig. 3-13).** It is often helpful to find a visual reference for the selected vein, such as a mole, freckle, or skin crease, to assist in relocating the vein after cleansing the site.

TECHNICAL TIP 3-16

According to CLSI standard GP41-A6 (H3-A6), an attempt should be made to locate the median cubital vein on both arms before considering other veins.

TECHNICAL TIP 3-17

Using the nondominant hand for palpation may be helpful when additional palpation is to be done immediately before performing the puncture.

TECHNICAL TIP 3-18

Leaving the alcohol pad on the arm below the venipuncture site, with the corner of the pad pointing to the insertion site, can be helpful in relocating veins that are not visible.

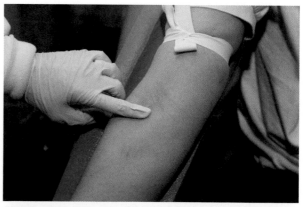

FIGURE 3-13 Palpating for a vein using the finger, not the thumb. *(Reproduced with permission from Strasinger, S.K., and Di Lorenzo, M.S.: The Phlebotomy Textbook, ed. 3. Philadelphia, F.A. Davis, 2011.)*

Many patients have prominent veins in one arm but not in the other arm. Checking the patient's other arm should be the first thing done when a site is not easily located. Patients with veins that are difficult to locate often point out areas of previously successful venipunctures. Palpation of these areas may prove beneficial and is also good for patient relations.

Other techniques to enhance the prominence of veins include massaging the arm upward from the wrist to the elbow, briefly hanging the arm down, and applying heat to the site for 3 to 5 minutes. A transilluminator device is helpful for locating veins, particularly in children. Tapping the site is not an acceptable technique because it can bruise the area, especially in an elderly patient. Remember that the tourniquet should not remain tied for more than 1 minute at a time when performing these techniques.

If no palpable veins are found in the antecubital area, the wrist and the back of the hand should be examined **(Fig. 3-14 A, B).** The tourniquet should be reapplied on the forearm. Because the veins in these areas are smaller, it may be necessary to change equipment and use a smaller needle with a syringe, a winged blood collection set, or a partial-draw evacuated tube.

⚠️ SAFETY TIP 3-10

CLSI standard GP41-A6 (H3-A6) cautions against selecting veins on the underside of the wrists to prevent nerve and tendon injuries.

TECHNICAL TIP 3-19

Never be reluctant to check both arms and to listen to the patient's suggestions. However, do not choose an inappropriate site based on the patient's request. A patient may not be aware of the dangers that could occur when drawing from those sites.

Veins in the legs, ankles, and feet should be used only with physician approval because of the potential for complications such as phlebitis, thrombosis, and tissue necrosis, particularly in patients with diabetes, cardiac problems, and coagulation disorders **(Fig. 3-15).**

Sites to Avoid

Certain areas must be avoided for venipuncture because of the possibility of decreased blood flow, infection, hemolysis, or sample contamination. Sites to avoid are listed in **Box 3-3**. Sample contamination affects the integrity of the sample, causing invalid tests results. Incorrect blood collection techniques that cause contamination include blood collected from edematous areas, blood collected from veins with hematomas, blood collected from arms containing an IV, sites contaminated with alcohol or iodine, or anticoagulant carryover between tubes.

Damaged Veins

Veins that contain thrombi or that have been subjected to numerous venipunctures often feel hard (sclerosed) and should be avoided because they may be blocked (occluded) and have impaired circulation.

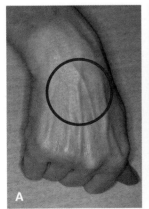
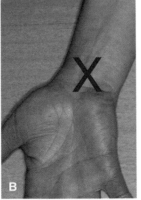

FIGURE 3-14 Alternative site for veinpuncture. *A,* **The back (posterior side) of the hand.** *B,* **Do NOT use the underside of the wrist.** *(Reproduced with permission from Strasinger, S.K., and Di Lorenzo, M.S.: The Phlebotomy Textbook, ed. 3. Philadelphia, F.A. Davis, 2011.)*

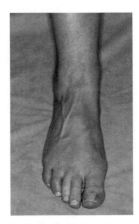

FIGURE 3-15 Veins in the foot. *(Reproduced with permission from Strasinger, S.K., and Di Lorenzo, M.S.: The Phlebotomy Textbook, ed. 3. Philadelphia, F.A. Davis, 2011.)*

BOX 3-3 Areas to Avoid for Venipuncture

Sclerosed veins
Occluded veins
Thrombosed veins
Hematomas
Edematous sites
Burned or scarred sites
Mastectomy side
Arm with an intravenous line
Heparin or saline locks
Arm with cannula or fistula

Areas that appear blue or are cold also may have impaired circulation.

Hematoma

The presence of a hematoma indicates that blood has accumulated in the tissue surrounding a vein **(Fig. 3-16)**. Puncturing into a hematoma not only is painful for the patient but also results in the collection of old hemolyzed blood from the hematoma rather than from circulating venous blood that is representative of the patient's current condition. If a vein containing a hematoma must be used, blood should be collected below the hematoma to ensure sampling of free-flowing blood.

Edema

Drawing from areas containing excess tissue fluid (edema) also is not recommended because the sample will be contaminated with tissue fluid. Edema may be caused by heart failure, renal failure, inflammation, or infection. Edema also may be caused by IV fluid infiltrating into the surrounding tissue.

Burns and Scars

Extensively burned and scarred areas are more susceptible to infection. They also have decreased circulation.

Mastectomy

Applying a tourniquet or drawing blood from an arm located on the same side of the body as a **mastectomy** can be harmful to the patient and produce erroneous test results. Removal of lymph nodes as part of the mastectomy procedure interferes with the flow of lymph fluid (lymphostasis) and increases the blood level of lymphocytes and waste products normally contained in the lymph fluid. Patients are in danger of developing lymphedema in the affected area. The protective functions of the lymphatic system are also lost, so that the area becomes more prone to infection. For these reasons, blood should be drawn from the other arm. In the case of a double mastectomy, the physician should be consulted as to an appropriate site. It may be possible to perform the tests from a finger stick but only with a physician's permission.

TECHNICAL TIP 3-20

Most mastectomy patients have been told never to have blood drawn from the affected side. Make sure they receive appropriate reassurance if an alternative site is not available and use of the affected side has been approved.

Obesity

Veins on obese patients are often deep and difficult to palpate. Often, the cephalic vein is more prominent. Using a syringe with a 1½-inch needle may offer more control.

IV Therapy

When a patient is receiving IV fluids, blood should be drawn from the other arm. When a patient has IVs in both arms, it is preferable to collect the sample by dermal puncture if possible. If an arm containing an IV must be used for sample collection, the site selected must be below the IV insertion point and preferably from a

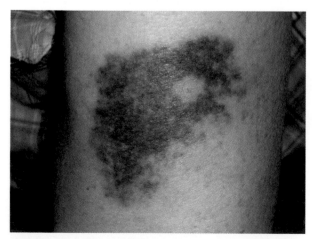

FIGURE 3-16 Hematoma formed from venipuncture. *(Reproduced with permission from Strasinger, S.K., and Di Lorenzo, M.S.: The Phlebotomy Textbook, ed. 3. Philadelphia, F.A. Davis, 2011.)*

different vein. The CLSI recommends having the nurse turn off the IV infusion for 2 minutes; the blood collector then may apply the tourniquet between the IV and the venipuncture site and perform the venipuncture. Document the location of the venipuncture (right or left arm) and that it was drawn below an infusion site. When blood is collected from an arm containing an IV, the type of fluid and location must be noted on the requisition form. Certain "add on tests" may not be acceptable from this sample. Avoid collecting blood too soon after dye for a radiological procedure has been injected or when a unit of blood is being infused.

TECHNICAL TIP 3-21

Inappropriate collection of blood from an arm containing an IV is a major cause of erroneous test results. Unless the sample is highly contaminated, the error may not be detected.

Heparin and Saline Locks

Heparin or saline locks are winged infusion sets connected to a stopcock or cap with a diaphragm that can be left in a vein for up to 48 hours to provide a means for administering frequently required medications and for obtaining blood samples. The devices must be flushed with heparin or saline periodically and after use to prevent blood clots from developing in the line. The first 5 mL of blood drawn must be discarded from either device. It is not recommended to collect blood through these devices for coagulation testing because residual heparin can affect test results.

SAFETY TIP 3-11

Only specifically trained personnel are authorized to draw blood from heparin and saline locks.

Cannulas and Fistulas

Patients receiving renal dialysis have a permanent surgical fusion of an artery and a vein called a fistula in one arm, and this arm should be avoided for venipuncture because of the possibility of infection. The dialysis patient also may have a temporary external connection between the artery and a vein formed by a cannula that

contains a special T-tube connector with a diaphragm for drawing blood. Only specifically trained personnel are authorized to draw blood from a cannula. Be sure to check for the presence of a fistula or cannula before applying a tourniquet to the arm, because this can compromise the patient. Accidental puncture of the area around the fistula can cause prolonged bleeding.

TECHNICAL TIP 3-22

Be alert for the presence of a fistula or cannula in dialysis patients before applying a tourniquet to the arm, because this can cause patient complications.

Cleanse the Site

After the vein is located, release the tourniquet and cleanse the site using a 70 percent isopropyl alcohol pad. Use a circular motion starting at the inside of the venipuncture site and work outward in widening concentric circles for 2 to 3 inches. Repeat this procedure for dirty skin. For maximum bacteriostatic action to occur, the alcohol should be allowed to dry for 30 to 60 seconds on the patient's arm rather than being wiped off with a gauze pad. The drying process helps kill the microorganisms. Performing a venipuncture before the alcohol has dried causes a stinging sensation for the patient and may hemolyze the sample. Do not reintroduce contaminants by blowing on the site, fanning the area, drying the site with unsterile gauze, or touching the site after cleansing it. If additional palpation of the vein is needed after the cleansing process, the blood collector should use alcohol to cleanse the gloved end of the finger to be used and touch only above or below the needle insertion point.

Blood cultures require that the site be cleansed with an antiseptic stronger than isopropyl alcohol. The most frequently used solutions are povidone-iodine, tincture of iodine, or chlorhexidine gluconate.

TECHNICAL TIP 3-23

Patients are quick to complain about a painful venipuncture. The stinging sensation caused by undried alcohol is a frequent, yet easily avoided, cause of a complaint.

Alcohol should not be used to cleanse the site prior to drawing a blood alcohol level. Thoroughly cleansing the site with soap and water ensures the least amount of interference, and some facilities find iodine or benzalkonium chloride (Zephiran Chloride) to be acceptable.

Assemble Puncture Equipment

While the alcohol is drying, make a final survey of the supplies at hand to be sure everything required for the procedure is present, and assemble the equipment.

Screw the stopper-puncturing end of the double-ended evacuated tube needle into the ETS holder. The needle and holder may come preassembled by the manufacturer. Do not remove the sterile colored cap from the other end of the needle. Insert the first tube to be collected into the tube holder up to the designated mark. After the tube is pushed up to the mark, it may retract slightly when pressure is released. This is acceptable.

 TECHNICAL TIP 3-24

Visual examination cannot detect all defective evacuated tubes; therefore, extra tubes should be at hand. It is not uncommon for the vacuum in a tube to be lost.

 TECHNICAL TIP 3-25

Place assembled venipuncture equipment within reach on the side of the blood collector's nondominant hand.

Perform the Venipuncture

Reapply the tourniquet and confirm the puncture site. If necessary, cleanse the gloved palpating finger for additional vein palpation. Ask the patient to again make a fist.

Examine the Needle

The ETS holder or syringe is held securely in the dominant hand with the thumb on top and the other fingers below. Before entering the vein, remove the needle's plastic cap and visually examine the point of the needle

for any defects, such as a bent or rough (barbed) end. Position the needle for entry into the vein with the bevel facing up.

Anchor the Vein

Use the thumb of the nondominant hand to anchor the selected vein while inserting the needle. Place the thumb 1 or 2 inches below and slightly to the side of the insertion site, and place the four fingers on the back of the arm and pull the skin taut. A vein that moves to the side is said to have "rolled." Patients often state that they have "rolling veins"; however, all veins will roll if they are not properly anchored. These patients are really saying that they have had blood drawn by practitioners who were not anchoring the veins well enough. As mentioned previously, the median cubital vein is the easiest to anchor and the basilic vein is the most difficult. In general, the closer a vein is to the surface, the more likely it is to roll.

Anchor hand veins by having the patient make a fist or grasp the end of a table or drawing chair arm. Pull the skin over the knuckles with the thumb of the nondominant hand.

 TECHNICAL TIP 3-26

Holding the tube holder or syringe in the position used for injections prevents threading the needle into the vein or bracing the hand for exchange of tubes.

 SAFETY TIP 3-12

Anchoring the vein above and below the site using the thumb and index finger is not an acceptable technique, because sudden patient movement could cause the index finger to be punctured.

Insert the Needle

When the vein is securely anchored, align the needle with the vein and insert it, bevel up, at an angle of 15 to 30 degrees depending on the depth of the vein. It should be done in a smooth, quick movement so that the patient feels the stick only briefly. You will notice a feeling of lessening of resistance to the needle movement when the vein has been entered. After needle insertion is made, the fingers are braced against the patient's arm to provide stability while tubes are being changed in the holder, or the plunger of the syringe is being pulled back.

TECHNICAL TIP 3-27

Tell the patient that "there will be a little stick" before needle insertion to alert the patient to hold very still.

TECHNICAL TIP 3-28

Entering the vein too slowly is more painful for the patient and may cause a spurt of blood to appear at the venipuncture site, which can be disconcerting for both the blood collector and patient.

Filling the Tubes

Once the vein has been entered, the hand anchoring the vein can be moved and used to push the evacuated tube completely into the holder or to pull back on the syringe plunger. Use the thumb to push the tube onto the back of the evacuated tube needle, while the index and middle fingers grasp the flared ends of the holder. Blood should begin to flow into the tube, and the tourniquet can be released by pulling the free end forward. Ask the patient to relax his or her fist.

The hand used to hold the needle assembly should remain braced on the patient's arm. This is of particular importance when evacuated tubes are being inserted or removed from the holder, because a certain amount of resistance is encountered and can cause the needle to be pushed through or pulled out of the vein. Tubes should be gently twisted on and off the puncturing needle using the flared ends of the holder as an additional brace.

To prevent any chance of blood refluxing back into the needle, tubes should be held at a downward angle while they are being filled and have slight pressure applied to them. Be sure to follow the prescribed order of draw when multiple tubes are being collected, and allow the tubes to fill completely before removing them. Mixing of evacuated tubes by gentle inversion for the correct number of times, depending on the anticoagulant or additive, should be done as soon as the tube is removed and before another tube is placed in the assembly. The few seconds required does not cause additional discomfort to the patient and ensures that the sample will be acceptable. Delay in mixing the sample may cause clots to form and necessitate recollecting the sample.

When the last tube has been filled, it is removed from the assembly and mixed prior to completing the procedure. Failure to remove the evacuated tube before removing the needle causes blood to drip from the end of the needle, resulting in unnecessary contamination and possible damage to the patient's clothes.

⚠️ SAFETY TIP 3-13

Pulling up or pressing down on the needle while it is in the vein can cause pain to the patient or a hematoma formation if blood leaks from the enlarged hole.

TECHNICAL TIP 3-29

Vigorous mixing of the sample can cause hemolysis and make the sample unacceptable for testing.

TECHNICAL TIP 3-30

Poor mixing may produce a sample with microclots that could yield erroneous test results.

Remove the Needle

Before removing the needle, remove the tourniquet if it is still on the patient. Failure to remove the tourniquet before removing the needle may produce a bruise or hematoma. Chapter 4 discusses other causes for hematoma formation.

TECHNICAL TIP 3-31

Allow tubes to fill until the vacuum is exhausted to ensure the correct blood-to-anticoagulant ratio.

Activate the needle safety device if it is designed to function while the needle is in the vein. Fold the gauze into fourths and place over the venipuncture site, smoothly withdraw the needle, and apply pressure to the site as soon as the needle is withdrawn. Do not apply pressure while the needle is still in the vein. Immediately activate the needle safety device if it is designed to function after the needle is removed from the vein.

To prevent blood from leaking into the surrounding tissue and producing a hematoma, pressure must be applied until the bleeding has stopped. The arm should be held in a raised, outstretched position. Bending the elbow to apply pressure allows blood to leak into the tissue more easily, causing a hematoma. A capable patient can be asked to apply the pressure, thereby freeing the blood collector to dispose of the used needle and label the sample tubes. If this is not possible, the blood collector must apply the pressure and perform the other tasks after the bleeding has stopped.

SAFETY TIP 3-14

CLSI standard GP41-A6 (H3-A6) recommends that the blood collector observe for hematoma formation by releasing pressure to the puncture and visually observing for subcutaneous bleeding before applying a bandage. Hematoma formation can place pressure on the nerves and cause a disabling compression nerve injury.

Disposal of the Contaminated Needle

On completion of the venipuncture, the contaminated needle with safety device activated must be disposed of immediately in an approved sharps container conveniently located near the patient. As discussed in Chapter 2, the method by which this is done depends on the type of disposal equipment selected by the facility. Under no circumstance should the needle be bent, cut, placed on a counter or bed, manually recapped, or removed from the tube holder after use.

SAFETY TIP 3-15

Needle safety devices must be activated immediately upon removal of the needle from the vein, whereas others must be activated while the needle is in the vein. Follow manufacturer's guidelines.

Label the Tubes

Tubes must be labeled at the time of sample collection, before leaving the patient's room or dismissing an outpatient. Tubes are labeled by writing with an indelible pen on the attached label or by applying a computer-generated label. Tubes should not be labeled before the sample is collected, because this can result in confusion of samples when more than one patient is having blood drawn or when a sample cannot be collected. Preprinted labels should be verified before being attached to the sample. Compare the labeled sample with the patient's ID band or request that the patient confirm that the tube is correctly labeled. Mislabeled samples, just like misidentified patients, can result in serious patient harm.

Information on the sample label should include the following:

- Patient's first and last name
- Patient's identification number (inpatient) or date of birth (outpatient)
- Date and time of collection
- Collector's initials

Additional information may be present on computer-generated labels. The laboratory will reject incompletely and unlabeled tubes. Samples for a blood bank test may require an additional label obtained from the patient's blood bank ID band.

Samples sent to the laboratory via a pneumatic tube system are placed in a biohazard bag. Samples requiring special handling, such as cooling or warming, are placed in the appropriate container when labeling is complete. (See Chapter 5.)

Bandage the Patient's Arm

Bleeding at the venipuncture site should stop within 5 minutes. Before applying the bandage, the blood collector should examine the patient's arm to be sure the bleeding has stopped. For additional pressure, an adhesive bandage or paper tape is applied over a folded-gauze square. A self-adhering, gauzelike material, such as a CoBan dressing, may be placed over the folded gauze and wrapped around the arm for patients with fragile skin or when additional pressure is needed. The patient should be instructed to remove the bandage after 15 minutes to avoid irritation and to avoid using the arm to carry heavy objects for 1 hour.

Patients receiving anticoagulant medications or large amounts of aspirin or herbs or patients with coagulation disorders may continue to bleed after pressure has been applied for 5 minutes. **Box 3-4** lists the herbs affecting coagulation testing. Continue to apply pressure until the bleeding has stopped.

In the case of an accidental arterial puncture, which usually can be detected by the appearance of unusually red blood that spurts into the tube, the blood collector, not the patient, should apply pressure to the site for 5 minutes or up to 10 minutes if the patient is on anticoagulant therapy. The fact that the sample is arterial blood should be recorded on the requisition form because some test values are different for arterial blood versus venous blood.

 SAFETY TIP 3-16

The practice of quickly applying tape over the gauze without checking the puncture site frequently produces hematomas.

Some patients are allergic to adhesive bandages, and it may be necessary to wrap gauze around the arm prior to applying the adhesive tape. Bandages are not recommended for children younger than 2 years old, because children may put bandages in their mouth.

Dispose of Used Supplies

Before leaving the patient's room, dispose of all contaminated supplies, such as alcohol, pads, and gauze, in a biohazard container; remove gloves and dispose of them in the biohazard container; and sanitize your hands. Needle caps and wrappers and other paper should be disposed of in the regular waste container.

Thank the Patient

Patients should be thanked for their cooperation in both inpatient and outpatient settings. Leave the patient's room in the condition in which you found it (bed and bedrails in the same position).

BOX 3-4 Herbs, Vitamins, and Dietary Supplements Having Effects on Coagulation and Blood Clotting

Garlic
Ginkgo biloba
Ginseng
Anise
Dong quai
Omega-3 fatty acids in fish oil
Ginger
Vitamin E
Fucus
Danshen
St. John's wort
Alfalfa
Coenzyme Q10
Bilberry
Bromelain
Cat's claw
Celery
Coleus
Cordyceps
Evening primrose
Fenugreek
Feverfew
Grape seed
Green tea
Guarana
Guggul
Horse chestnut seed
Horseradish
Horsetail rush
Licorice
Prickly ash
Red clover
Reishi
Sweet clover
Turmeric
White willow

Reproduced with permission from Strasinger, S.K., and Di Lorenzo, M.S.: The Phlebotomy Textbook, ed. 3. Philadelphia, F.A. Davis, 2011.

Deliver Samples to the Laboratory

Deliver each sample to the laboratory as soon as possible. Gently transport samples in a vertical position to facilitate clotting and prevent hemolysis. Use designated biohazard containers for transport **(Fig. 3-17),** and securely attach the requisitions with the sample when using the pneumatic tube system. Perform the correct wrapping of the sample to avoid breakage and verify that the pneumatic tube has been sent before leaving. Follow procedures for samples requiring special handling, which are covered in Chapter 5.

Sample Processing

The stability of analytes varies greatly, as do the accepted methods of preservation. This is why rapid delivery to the laboratory or following laboratory-prescribed sample-handling protocols is essential. Common protocols include separation of the plasma or serum from the cells (either manually or by gel), storage temperature, and protection of the sample from exposure to light. Gel separation tubes must always be stored in an upright position.

The CLSI recommends centrifugation of tubes and the separation of plasma or serum from the cells within 2 hours. Ideally, the sample should reach the laboratory within 45 minutes and be centrifuged on arrival. Tests most frequently affected by improper processing include glucose, potassium, and coagulation tests. Glycolysis caused by the use of glucose in cellular metabolism causes falsely lower glucose values. Hemolysis and leakage of intracellular potassium into the serum or plasma falsely elevates potassium results. According to the CLSI guidelines, coagulation samples for activated partial thromboplastin times (APTTs) are stable at room temperature for 4 hours unless the patient is on heparin, in which case the plasma must be removed from the cells within 1 hour after collection and tested

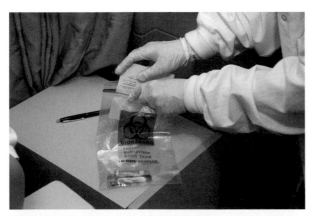

FIGURE 3-17 Placing sample and requisition in a biohazard bag for transporting. *(Reproduced with permission from Strasinger, S.K., and Di Lorenzo, M.S.: The Phlebotomy Textbook, ed. 3. Philadelphia, F.A. Davis, 2011.)*

within 4 hours. Samples for prothrombin time (PT) testing are stable for 24 hours at room temperature. All other coagulation tests must be performed within 4 hours of collection. When samples cannot be assayed within the required time frame, the platelet-poor plasma must be separated from the red cells and frozen within 1 hour of collection. Appendix A summarizes the requirements of some routinely encountered analytes.

The venipuncture procedure is complete when the sample is delivered to the laboratory in satisfactory condition and all appropriate paperwork has been completed. These procedures vary, depending on facility protocol and the types of samples collected. The routine venipuncture procedure using the evacuated tube system is illustrated in **Procedure 3-2.**

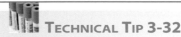

TECHNICAL TIP 3-32

Verification of the sample collection either into the computer or recorded in a logbook completes the collection process.

Using a Syringe

Although the evacuated tubes system is the recommended procedure for blood collection, it may be necessary to use a syringe to better control the pressure applied to the delicate veins found in pediatric and elderly patients, or when drawing from hand veins.

Except for a few minor differences, the procedure for drawing blood using a syringe is the same as when using an ETS. Blood is withdrawn from the vein by slowly pulling on the plunger of the syringe using the hand that is free after the anchored vein is entered. The advantage of using a syringe is that when the vein is entered, blood will appear in the hub of the needle and the plunger can then be pulled back at a speed that corresponds to the rate of blood flow into the syringe. Pulling the plunger back faster than the rate of blood flow may cause the walls of the vein to collapse and can cause hemolysis. Pulling the plunger back too slowly may cause the blood to begin to clot in the syringe before the blood is collected and transferred to anticoagulated tubes. It is important to anchor the hand holding the syringe firmly on the patient's arm so that the needle will not move when the plunger is pulled.

(Text continued on page 73)

PROCEDURE 3-2 **Venipuncture Using an Evacuated Tube System**

EQUIPMENT:

Requisition form	Evacuated tubes
Gloves	2 × 2 gauze
Tourniquet	Sharps container
70 percent isopropyl alcohol pad	Indelible pen
Evacuated tube needle with safety device	Bandage
Evacuated tube holder with safety device if the needle does not have one	Biohazard bag

PROCEDURE:

Step 1. Obtain and examine the requisition form.

Step 2. Greet and reassure the patient and explain the procedure to be performed. Obtain patient informed consent.

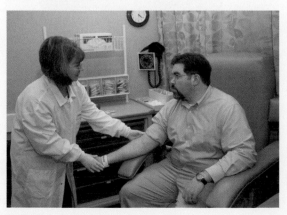

Step 3. Identify the patient verbally by having him or her state both the first name and last name and compare the information on the patient's ID band with the requisition form.

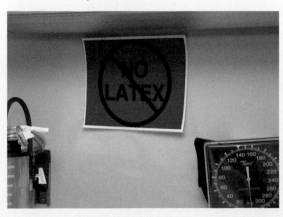

Step 4. Verify whether the patient has fasted, has allergies to latex, or has had previous problems with venipuncture.

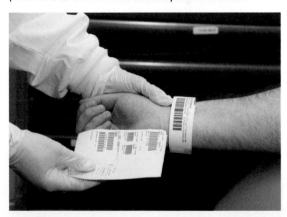

Step 5. Select correct tubes and equipment for the procedure. Have extra tubes available.

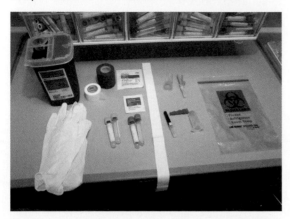

Step 6. Sanitize hands and apply gloves.

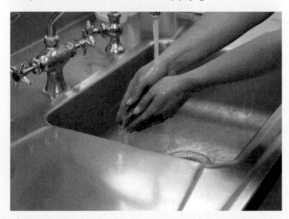

Step 7. Position the patient's arm slightly bent in a downward position so that the tubes fill from the bottom up. Do not allow blood to touch the stopper-puncturing needle. Do not let the patient hyperextend the arm. Ask the patient to make a fist.

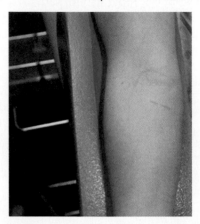

Step 8. Apply the tourniquet 3 to 4 inches above the antecubital fossa. Palpate the area in a vertical and horizontal direction to locate a large vein and to determine the depth, direction, and size. The median cubital is the vein of choice, followed by the cephalic vein. The basilic vein should be avoided if possible. Remove the tourniquet and have the patient open his or her fist.

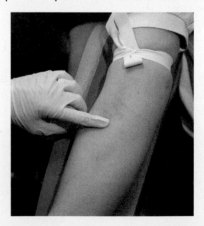

PROCEDURE 3-2 Venipuncture Using an Evacuated Tube System (Continued)

Step 9. Clean the sie with 70 percent isopropyl alcohol in concentric circles moving outward and allow it to air-dry.

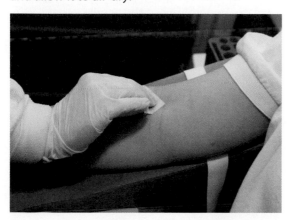

Step 11. Insert the tube into the holder up to the tube advancement mark.

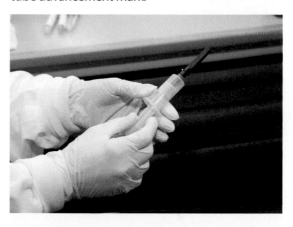

Step 10. Assemble the equipment while the alcohol is drying. Attach the multi-sample needle to the holder.

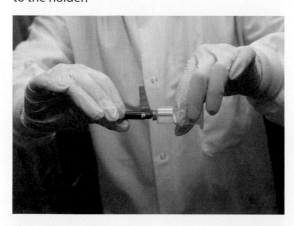

Step 12. Reapply the tourniquet. Do not touch the puncture site with an unclean finger. Ask the patient to remake a fist. Patient should be instructed not to "pump" or "continuously clench" the fist to prevent hemoconcentration.

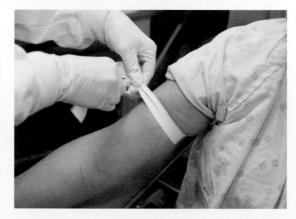

PROCEDURE 3-2 Venipuncture Using an Evacuated Tube System (Continued)

Step 13. Remove the plastic needle cap and examine the needle for defects such as nonpointed or barbed ends.

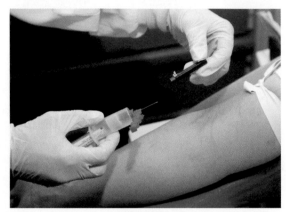

Step 14. Anchor the vein by placing the thumb of the nondominant hand 1 to 2 inches below the site and pulling the skin taut.

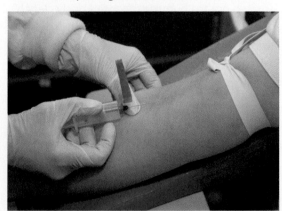

Step 15. Grasp the assembled needle and tube holder using your dominant hand with the thumb on the top near the hub and your other fingers beneath. Smoothly insert the needle into the vein at a 15- to 30-degree angle with the bevel up until you feel a lessening of resistance. Brace the fingers against the arm to prevent movement of the needle when changing tubes.

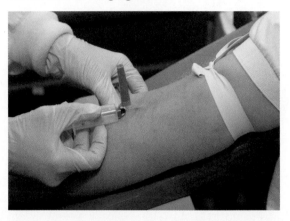

Step 16. Using the thumb, advance the tube on to the evacuated tube needle, while the index and middle fingers grasp the flared ends of the holder.

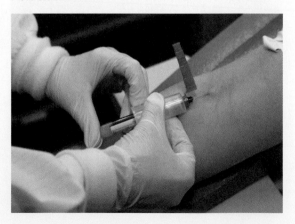

PROCEDURE 3-2 **Venipuncture Using an Evacuated Tube System** (Continued)

Step 17. When blood flows into the tube, release the tourniquet and ask the patient to open the fist.

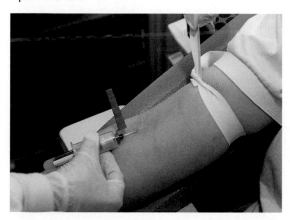

Step 18. Gently remove the tube when the blood stops flowing into it. Gently invert anti-coagulated tubes promptly. Insert the next tube using the correct order of draw. Fill tubes completely.

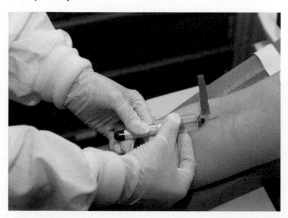

Step 19. Remove the last tube collected from the holder and gently invert.

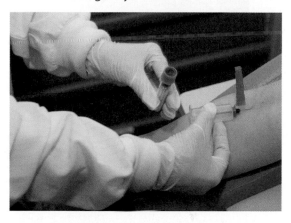

Step 20. Cover the puncture site with clean gauze. Remove the needle smoothly and apply pressure or ask the patient to apply pressure.

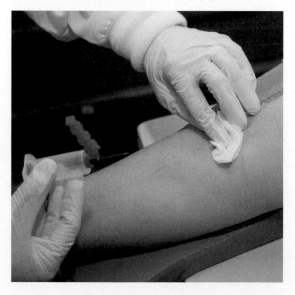

PROCEDURE 3-2   Venipuncture Using an Evacuated Tube System (Continued)

Step 21. Activate the safety device.

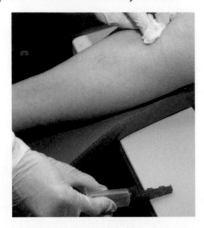

Step 22. Dispose the needle/holder assembly with the safety device activated into the sharps container.

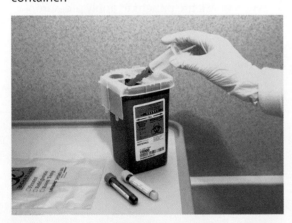

Step 23. Label the tubes before leaving the patient and verify identification with the patient ID band or verbally with an outpatient. Observe any special handling procedures. Complete paperwork.

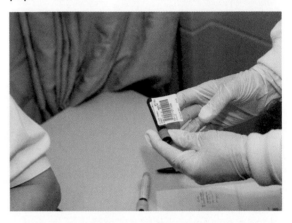

Step 24. Examine the puncture site and apply bandage. Place bandage over folded gauze for additional pressure.

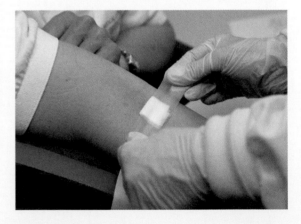

PROCEDURE 3-2 **Venipuncture Using an Evacuated Tube System** (Continued)

Step 25. Prepare sample and requisition for transportation to the laboratory. Dispose of used supplies.

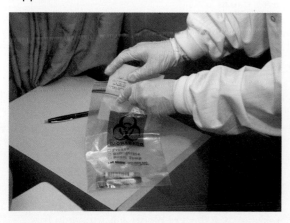

Modified with permission from Strasinger, S.K., and Di Lorenzo, M.S.: The Phlebotomy Textbook, ed. 3. Philadelphia, F.A. Davis, 2011.

Step 26. Thank the patient, remove gloves, and sanitize hands.

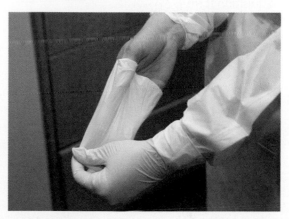

Ideally, the size of the syringe used should correspond to the amount of blood needed. It may be necessary to fill two or more smaller syringes when veins are small and may easily collapse. This will require assistance, because blood from the filled syringe must be transferred to the appropriate tubes while the second syringe is being filled. It is important that blood be added to anticoagulated tubes as soon as possible. Before exchanging syringes, gauze must be placed on the patient's arm under the needle because blood will leak from the hub of the needle during the exchange.

As discussed in Chapter 2, blood is transferred from the syringe to evacuated tubes, following the correct order of fill, using a blood transfer device. After removing the needle from the vein, activate the needle safety device and remove the needle and discard it in the sharps container. The blood transfer device is attached to the syringe and evacuated tubes are pushed on to the stopper-puncturing rubber-sheathed needle. After the tubes are filled, the syringe and blood transfer device are discarded into a sharps container. The venipuncture procedure using a syringe is shown in **Procedure 3-3.**

 TECHNICAL TIP 3-33

In most circumstances, the use of small evacuated tubes with a winged blood collection set instead of a syringe can prevent the need to change syringes.

⚠ **SAFETY TIP 3-17**

Pushing on the plunger can hemolyze the red blood cells or cause the tube stopper to pop off, risking an aerosol spray.

 TECHNICAL TIP 3-34

Transfer the blood quickly from the syringe to the evacuated tube to avoid the possibility of the blood clotting. Do not lay the syringe aside to complete the venipuncture procedure before transferring the blood.

PROCEDURE 3-3 Venipuncture Using a Syringe

EQUIPMENT:

Requisition form
Gloves
Tourniquet
70 percent isopropyl alcohol pad
Syringe needle with safety device
Syringe
Blood transfer device

Evacuated tubes
2 × 2 gauze
Sharps container
Indelible pen
Bandage
Biohazard bag

PROCEDURE:

Step 1. Perform steps 1 to 9 of Procedure 3-2, "Venipuncture Using an Evacuated Tube System."

Step 2. Assemble the equipment as the alcohol is drying. Attach the hypodermic needle to the syringe. Pull the plunger back to ensure that it moves freely and then push it forward to remove any air in the syringe.

Step 3. Reapply the tourniquet, remove the needle cap, and inspect the needle.

Step 4. Ask the patient to remake a fist, and anchor the vein by placing the thumb of the non-dominant hand 1 to 2 inches below the site and pulling the skin taut.

Step 5. Hold the syringe in the dominant hand with the thumb on top near the hub and the other fingers underneath. Smoothly insert the needle into the vein at a 15- to 30-degree angle with the bevel up until you feel a lessening of resistance. A flash of blood will appear in the syringe hub when the vein has been entered. Brace the fingers against the arm to prevent movement of the needle when pulling back on the plunger.

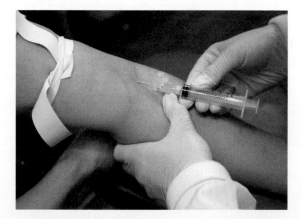

PROCEDURE 3-3 Venipuncture Using a Syringe (Continued)

Step 6. Pull back the syringe plunger slowly using the nondominant hand to collect the appropriate amount of blood.

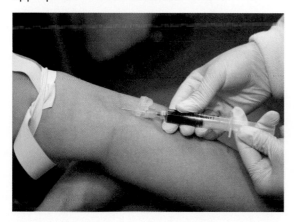

Step 7. Release the tourniquet and have the patient open the fist.

Step 8. Cover the puncture site with gauze, remove the needle smoothly, activate the safety device, and apply pressure.

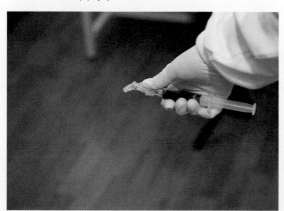

Step 9. Remove the needle from the syringe and discard it in the sharps container.

Step 10. Attach a blood transfer device to the syringe.

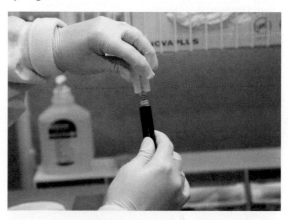

Step 11. Holding the syringe vertically with the blood transfer device at the bottom, advance the evacuated tube on to the internal needle in the blood transfer device. Tubes will fill by the vacuum in the tube. Keep the tube in a vertical position to ensure that the tubes fill from the bottom up to avoid cross-contamination. Do not push on the plunger.

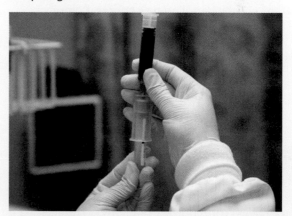

PROCEDURE 3-3 Venipuncture Using a Syringe (Continued)

Step 12. Fill tubes in the correct order. Mix anticoagulated tubes as soon as they are removed from the transfer device.

Step 13. After tubes are filled, the entire syringe and blood transfer device are discarded into a sharps container.

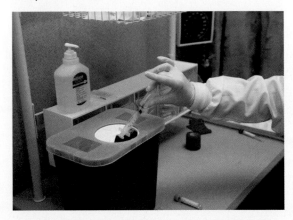

Step 14. Label the tubes before leaving the patient and verify identification with the patient ID band or verbally with an outpatient. Observe any special handling procedures. Complete paperwork.

Modified with permission from Strasinger, S.K., and Di Lorenzo, M.S.: The Phlebotomy Textbook, ed. 3. Philadelphia, F.A. Davis, 2011.

Step 15. Examine the puncture site and apply bandage. Place bandage over folded gauze for additional pressure.

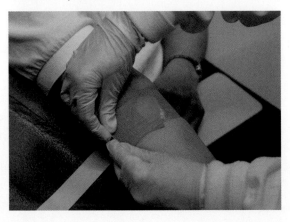

Step 16. Prepare sample and requisition for transportation to the laboratory. Dispose of used supplies.

Step 17. Thank the patient, remove gloves, and sanitize hands.

Using a Winged Blood Collection Set

All routine venipuncture procedures used with evacuated tubes and syringes also apply to blood collection using a winged blood collection set (butterfly). This method is used for difficult venipuncture and is often less painful to patients. The angle of needle insertion can be lowered to 10 to 15 degrees, facilitating entry into small veins by folding the plastic needle attachments ("wings") upward while inserting the needle. Blood will appear in the tubing when the vein is entered. The needle can then be threaded securely into the vein and kept in place by holding the plastic wings against the patient's arm.

Depending on the type of winged blood collection set used, blood can be collected into an evacuated tube or a syringe. The tubing contains a small amount of air (0.5 mL) that will cause underfilling of the first tube; therefore, a discard tube should be collected before a coagulation tube to prime the line and maintain the correct blood-to-anticoagulant ratio.

To prevent hemolysis when using a small (23-gauge) needle, partial-draw evacuated tubes should be used. Tubes are positioned downward to fill from the bottom up and in the same order of draw as in evacuated tube venipuncture. If blood has been collected into a syringe, the winged blood collection needle safety device is activated and removed from the syringe. A blood transfer device is attached to the syringe and the evacuated tubes are filled in the correct order.

SAFETY TIP 3-18

When using a winged blood collection set, be sure to attach the holder to the stopper-puncturing needle and not just push the tubes on to the back of the rubber sheathed needle. This will avoid an accidental needle-stick exposure from the stopper-puncturing needle.

When disposing of the winged blood collection set, use extreme care, because many accidental sticks result from unexpected movement of the tubing. Immediately activating the needle safety device and placing the needle into a sharps container and then allowing the tubing to fall into the container when the evacuated tube or syringe is removed can prevent accidents. Using an apparatus with automatic resheathing capability or activating a device on the needle set that advances a safety blunt before removing the needle from the vein is recommended to prevent accidental needle punctures. Do not push the apparatus manually into a full sharps container.

SAFETY TIP 3-19

Always hold a winged blood collection set by the wings, not by the tubing.

The venipuncture procedure using a winged blood collection set is shown in **Procedure 3-4.**

PROCEDURE 3-4 Venipuncture Using a Winged Blood Collection Set

EQUIPMENT:

Requisition form	Evacuated tubes
Gloves	2 × 2 gauze
Tourniquet	Sharps container
70 percent isopropyl alcohol pad	Indelible pen
Winged blood collection set	Bandage
Syringe or ETS holder	Biohazard bag
Blood transfer device	

PROCEDURE:

Step 1. Perform steps 1 to 6 of Procedure 3-2, "Venipuncture Using an Evacuated Tube System."

Step 2. Support the hand on the bed or drawing chair armrest and have the patient make a loose fist.

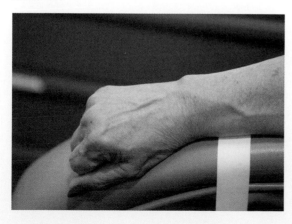

Step 3. Apply the tourniquet 3 to 4 inches above the wrist bone.

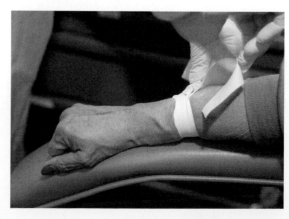

PROCEDURE 3-4 Venipuncture Using a Winged Blood Collection Set (Continued)

Step 4. Palpate the top of the hand or wrist. Select a vein that is large and straight and that can be easily anchored.

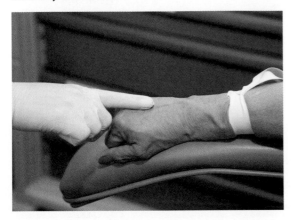

Step 5. Release the tourniquet, have the patient relax the fist, and clean the site with 70 percent isopropyl alcohol in concentric circles and allow to air-dry.

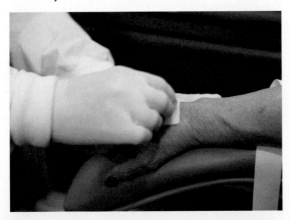

Step 6. Assemble the equipment as the alcohol is drying. Attach the winged blood collection set to the evacuated tube holder or the syringe. Stretch out the coiled tubing. Pull the plunger back to ensure that it moves freely and then push it forward to remove any air in the syringe. If using an evacuated tube holder, insert the first tube to the tube advancement mark.

Step 7. Reapply the tourniquet, remove the needle cap, and inspect the needle. Lay the syringe and tubing next to the patient's hand.

Step 8. Anchor the vein by placing the thumb of the nondominant hand below the knuckles and pulling the skin taut. Having the patient make a loose fist may be helpful.

Step 9. Grasp the needle between the thumb and index finger by holding the back of the needle or by folding the wings together. Smoothly insert the needle into the vein at a shallow 10- to 15-degree angle with the bevel up. Thread the needle into the lumen of the vein until the bevel is firmly "seated" in the vein. A flash of blood will appear in the tubing when the needle has entered the vein.

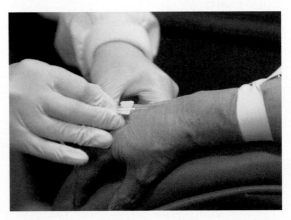

PROCEDURE 3-4 **Venipuncture Using a Winged Blood Collection Set** (Continued)

Step 10. Pull back on the plunger of the syringe slowly and smoothly with the nondominant hand to collect blood. Do not pull back on the syringe plunger if a blood flash does not appear. When using an evacuated tube holder, insert the tubes in the correct order of draw. Use a discard tube when collecting anticoagulated tubes to prime the tubing and maintain the correct blood-to-anticoagulant ratio. Invert anticoagulated tubes immediately.

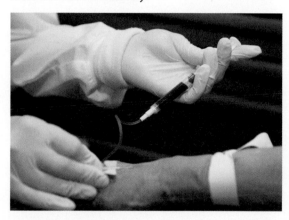

Step 11. Release the tourniquet.

Step 12. Cover the puncture site with gauze, remove the needle smoothly or activate the safety device on needles designed to be retracted while the needle is in the vein.

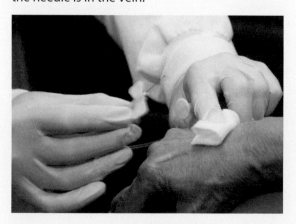

Step 13. Activate the safety device for needles designed to be shielded when the needle is out of the vein, and apply pressure.

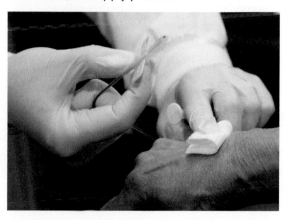

Step 14. Remove the winged blood collection set from the syringe and discard it in the sharps container.

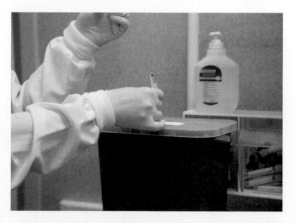

Step 15. Attach a blood transfer device to the syringe and fill the evacuated tubes in the correct order.

Step 16. After tubes are filled, the syringe and blood transfer device are discarded into a sharps container.

PROCEDURE 3-4 Venipuncture Using a Winged Blood Collection Set (Continued)

Step 17. Label the tubes before leaving the patient and verify identification with the patient ID band or verbally with an outpatient. Observe any special handling procedures. Complete paperwork.

Step 18. Examine the puncture site and apply a bandage. Place bandage over folded gauze for additional pressure.

Step 19. Prepare sample and requisition for transportation to the laboratory. Dispose of used supplies.

Step 20. Thank the patient, remove gloves, and sanitize hands.

Modified with permission from Strasinger, S.K., and Di Lorenzo, M.S.: The Phlebotomy Textbook, ed. 3. Philadelphia, F.A. Davis, 2011.

BIBLIOGRAPHY

CLSI: *Procedures for the Collection of Diagnostic Blood Specimens by Venipuncture*, ed. 6. Approved Guideline GP41-A6 (H03-A6). Wayne, PA, CLSI, 2007.

CLSI: *Collection, Transport, and Processing of Blood Specimens for Testing Plasma-Based Coagulation Assays and Molecular Hemostasis Assays*, ed. 2 Approved Standard H21-A5. Wayne, PA, CLSI, 2012.

CLSI: *Procedures for the Handling and Processing of Blood Specimens for Common Laboratory Tests*, ed. 4, Approved Guideline GP44-A4 (H18-A4). Wayne, PA, CLSI, 2012.

Strasinger, S.K., and DiLorenzo, M.S.: *The Phlebotomy Textbook*, ed. 3. Philadelphia, F.A. Davis, 2011.

INTERNET RESOURCES

www.clsi.org

www.jointcommission.org

www.bd.com/vacutainer/labnotes

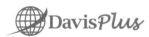 For additional material, please visit http://davisplus.fadavis .com.

REVIEW QUESTIONS

1. The most important step in the venipuncture procedure is:
   a. Applying the tourniquet
   b. Locating the best vein
   c. Identifying the patient
   d. Applying pressure to the puncture site

2. The minimum number of patient identifiers required by The Joint Commission is:
   a. 1
   b. 2
   c. 3
   d. 4

3. To avoid interference with test results, the maximum time that a tourniquet can remain on the patient's arm is:
   a. 1 minute
   b. 2 minutes
   c. 5 minutes
   d. 10 minutes

4. The venipuncture step of primary importance to prevent rolling veins is:
   a. Tightly applying the tourniquet
   b. Selecting the median cubital vein
   c. Using a 23-gauge needle
   d. Anchoring the vein while inserting the needle

5. Which of the following areas can be used for venipuncture?
   a. The deep cephalic vein
   b. From a hematoma
   c. An arm with an IV running
   d. An arm with a fistula

6. The needle is inserted into the vein:
   a. Bevel up at a 45- to 50-degree angle
   b. Bevel up at a 15- to 30-degree angle
   c. Bevel down at a 15- to 30-degree angle
   d. Bevel down at a 45- to 50-degree angle

7. If the plunger of a syringe is pulled back too fast:
   a. The patient will develop a hematoma
   b. The patient feels a stinging sensation
   c. Excess needle movement is prevented
   d. The sample may be hemolyzed

8. Which of the following is the proper procedure to avoid a hematoma?
   a. Removing the tourniquet after removing the needle
   b. Bandaging the patient's arm immediately after needle removal
   c. Firmly anchoring the vein in needle insertion
   d. Having the patient bend the elbow and apply pressure

9. Prior to bandaging the puncture site, the blood collector should:
   a. Thank the patient
   b. Instruct a fasting patient to eat
   c. Examine the site for bleeding
   d. Apply pressure for at least 5 minutes

10. When collecting blood using a winged blood collection set with a 23-gauge needle, which of the following is acceptable:
    a. Raising the angle of insertion to 45 degrees
    b. Collecting blood into a syringe
    c. Using a 15-mL evacuated tube
    d. Filling the SST tube before the light blue stopper tube

FOR FURTHER STUDY

1. Determine whether the following are acceptable or not acceptable when performing a venipuncture, and explain your reason in one sentence.
   a. An outpatient with a sore back wanting to stand during the procedure.
   b. Assembling equipment before applying the tourniquet.
   c. Requesting the patient to pump his or her fist during sample collection.
   d. Cleansing the site in a circular motion from inside to outside.
   e. Bending the patient's elbow while applying pressure to the puncture site.

2. State an error in routine venipuncture technique that may cause:
   a. A hematoma
   b. Petechiae
   c. A patient to choke
   d. Blood to stop flowing when a tube is changed
   e. Blood drops on a patient's slacks when the needle is removed

3. List three reasons for vein palpation.

4. State two errors in test results that can be caused by prolonged tourniquet application.

CASE STUDY 3-1

Sandra worked in a busy internal medicine clinic that specialized in infectious diseases and that required all patients to have blood drawn for detection of HIV, hepatitis B virus (HBV), and hepatitis C virus (HCV) at each visit. Sandra quickly called Mary back to the drawing station using her first name. Sandra immediately applied the tourniquet, selected a vein, assembled the equipment, labeled the tubes, cleansed the site, blew on the site to dry the alcohol, and performed the venipuncture.

1. What is wrong with this situation?

2. State three ways in which the patient, the blood collector, or sample in this scenario could be affected.

3. What legal ramifications may be possible?

CASE STUDY 3-2

Monica enters the diagnostic center for follow-up laboratory tests. After proper identification, she states that she had a mastectomy 3 months ago. She holds her left arm out for the blood collection.

1. What question(s) should the blood collector ask Monica?

2. If blood is drawn from the wrong arm, state two possible dangers to Monica.

3. If blood is drawn from the wrong arm, state two possible effects on the laboratory tests.

EVALUATION OF TOURNIQUET APPLICATION AND VEIN SELECTION

RATING SYSTEM:

2 = Satisfactory

1 = Needs improvement

0 = Incorrect/did not perform

_____ 1. Positions arm correctly for vein selection.

_____ 2. Selects appropriate tourniquet application site.

_____ 3. Places tourniquet in flat position behind arm.

_____ 4. Smoothly positions hands when crossing and tucking tourniquet.

_____ 5. Fastens tourniquet at appropriate tightness.

_____ 6. Tourniquet is not folded into arm.

_____ 7. Loop and loose end do not interfere with puncture site.

_____ 8. Asks patient to clench fist.

_____ 9. Selects antecubital area to palpate.

_____ 10. Performs palpation using correct fingers.

_____ 11. Palpates entire area or both arms if necessary.

_____ 12. Checks size, depth, and direction of veins.

_____ 13. Removes tourniquet smoothly.

_____ 14. Removes tourniquet in a timely manner.

TOTAL POINTS

MAXIMUM POINTS = 28

COMMENTS:

EVALUATION OF VENIPUNCTURE TECHNIQUE USING AN EVACUATED TUBE SYSTEM

RATING SYSTEM:

2 = Satisfactory

1 = Needs improvement

0 = Incorrect/did not perform

_____ 1. Examines requisition form.

_____ 2. Greets patient and states procedure to be done.

_____ 3. Obtains patient informed consent.

_____ 4. Identifies patient verbally.

_____ 5. Examines patient's ID band.

_____ 6. Compares requisition information with ID band.

_____ 7. Selects correct tubes and equipment for procedure.

_____ 8. Sanitizes hands and puts on gloves.

_____ 9. Positions patient's arm.

_____ 10. Applies tourniquet.

_____ 11. Identifies vein by palpation.

_____ 12. Releases tourniquet.

_____ 13. Cleanses site and allows it to air-dry.

_____ 14. Assembles equipment and conveniently places equipment.

_____ 15. Reapplies tourniquet.

_____ 16. Does not touch puncture site with unclean finger.

_____ 17. Removes needle cap and examines needle.

_____ 18. Anchors vein below puncture site.

_____ 19. Smoothly enters vein at appropriate angle with bevel up.

_____ 20. Does not move needle when changing tubes.

_____ 21. Collects tubes in correct order.

_____ 22. Mixes anticoagulated tubes promptly.

_____ 23. Fills tubes completely.

_____ 24. Releases tourniquet within 1 minute.

_____ 25. Removes last tube collected from holder.

_____ 26. Covers puncture site with gauze.

_____ 27. Removes the needle smoothly and applies pressure.

_____ 28. Activates needle safety device.

_____ 29. Disposes of the needle in sharps container with safety device activated and attached to the holder.

_____ 30. Labels tubes.

_____ 31. Confirms labeled tube by comparing it with the patient ID band or has patient verify that the information is correct.

_____ 32. Examines puncture site.

_____ 33. Applies bandage.

_____ 34. Disposes of used supplies.

_____ 35. Removes gloves and sanitizes hands.

_____ 36. Thanks patient.

_____ 37. Converses appropriately with patient during procedure.

TOTAL POINTS

MAXIMUM POINTS = 74

COMMENTS:

EVALUATION OF VENIPUNCTURE TECHNIQUE USING A SYRINGE

RATING SYSTEM

2 = Satisfactory

1 = Needs improvement

0 = Incorrect/did not perform

_____ 1. Examines requisition form.

_____ 2. Greets patient and states procedure to be done.

_____ 3. Obtains patient informed consent.

_____ 4. Identifies patient verbally.

_____ 5. Examines patient's ID band.

_____ 6. Compares requisition form with ID band.

_____ 7. Selects tubes and equipment for procedure.

_____ 8. Sanitizes hands and puts on gloves.

_____ 9. Positions patient's arm.

_____ 10. Applies tourniquet.

_____ 11. Identifies vein by palpation.

_____ 12. Releases tourniquet.

_____ 13. Cleanses site and allows it to air-dry.

_____ 14. Assembles and conveniently places equipment.

_____ 15. Reapplies tourniquet.

_____ 16. Does not touch puncture site with unclean finger.

_____ 17. Checks plunger movement.

_____ 18. Removes needle cap and examines needle.

_____ 19. Anchors vein below puncture site.

_____ 20. Smoothly enters vein at appropriate angle with bevel up.

_____ 21. Does not move needle when plunger is retracted.

_____ 22. Collects appropriate amount of blood.

_____ 23. Releases tourniquet.

_____ 24. Covers puncture site with gauze.

_____ 25. Removes needle smoothly, activates the safety device, and applies pressure.

_____ 26. Uses a blood transfer device to fill tubes.

_____ 27. Fills tubes in correct order.

_____ 28. Mixes anticoagulated tubes promptly.

_____ 29. Disposes of needle, transfer device, and syringe in sharps container.

_____ 30. Labels tubes.

_____ 31. Confirms labeled tube by comparing it with the patient ID band or has patient verify that the information is correct.

_____ 32. Examines puncture site.

_____ 33. Applies bandage.

_____ 34. Disposes of used supplies.

_____ 35. Removes gloves and sanitizes hands.

_____ 36. Thanks patient.

_____ 37. Converses appropriately with patient during procedure.

TOTAL POINTS

MAXIMUM POINTS = 74

COMMENTS:

EVALUATION OF VENIPUNCTURE TECHNIQUE USING A WINGED BLOOD COLLECTION SET

RATING SYSTEM:

2 = Satisfactory

1 = Needs improvement

0 = Incorrect/did not perform

_____ 1. Examines requisition form.

_____ 2. Greets patient and states procedure to be done.

_____ 3. Obtains patient's informed consent.

_____ 4. Identifies patient verbally.

_____ 5. Examines patient's ID band.

_____ 6. Compares requisition form with ID band.

_____ 7. Selects tubes and equipment for procedure.

_____ 8. Sanitizes hands and puts on gloves.

_____ 9. Positions patient's hand.

_____ 10. Applies tourniquet.

_____ 11. Identifies vein by palpation.

_____ 12. Releases tourniquet.

_____ 13. Cleanses site and allows it to air-dry.

_____ 14. Assembles and conveniently places equipment.

_____ 15. Reapplies tourniquet.

_____ 16. Does not touch puncture site with unclean finger.

_____ 17. Checks plunger movement if a syringe is attached.

_____ 18. Removes needle cap and examines needle.

_____ 19. Anchors vein below puncture site.

_____ 20. Holds needle appropriately.

_____ 21. Enters vein smoothly at appropriate angle with bevel up.

_____ 22. Maintains needle securely in vein.

_____ 23. Smoothly operates syringe or evacuated tube holder.

_____ 24. Fills tubes in the correct order.

_____ 25. Mixes anticoagulated tubes promptly.

_____ 26. Collects appropriate amount of blood.

_____ 27. Releases tourniquet.

_____ 28. Covers puncture site with gauze.

_____ 29. Removes needle smoothly, activates safety device, and applies pressure.

_____ 30. Disposes of apparatus in sharps container.

_____ 31. Uses a blood transfer device to fill tubes in the correct order when syringe is attached.

_____ 32. Labels tubes.

_____ 33. Confirms labeled tube by comparing it with the patient ID band or has patient verify that the information is correct.

_____ 34. Examines puncture site.

_____ 35. Applies bandage.

_____ 36. Disposes of used supplies.

_____ 37. Removes gloves and sanitizes hands.

_____ 38. Thanks patient.

_____ 39. Converses appropriately with patient during procedure.

TOTAL POINTS

MAXIMUM POINTS = 78

COMMENTS:

Preexamination Variables and Venipuncture Complications

LEARNING OBJECTIVES

Upon completion of this chapter, the reader will be able to:

4.1 Discuss the preexamination variables related to blood collection that can affect the quality of laboratory tests and patient outcomes.

4.2 Describe technical complications related to blood collection and the remedies for each situation.

4.3 List the reasons blood may not be immediately obtained from a venipuncture and the procedures to follow to obtain blood.

4.4 List six causes of hematomas.

4.5 Discuss the venipuncture errors that may produce hemolysis.

4.6 Explain five causes of sample contamination.

4.7 Discuss patient complications and an effective method to handle each situation.

4.8 Identify the specific requirements related to blood collection in the geriatric and pediatric populations.

4.9 List five reasons for rejecting a sample.

KEY TERMS

Basal State Metabolic condition after 12 hours of fasting and lack of exercise

Compartment Syndrome Blood accumulates within the tissues of the muscles that surround the arm or hand and causes increased pressure in the area

Diurnal Variation Normal changes in blood constituent levels at different times of the day

Fasting Abstinence from food and liquids (except water) for a specified period

Geriatric Pertaining to old age

Hematoma Discoloration of the skin (bruise) produced by the leakage of blood into the tissue

Hemolysis Destruction of red blood cells

Iatrogenic Pertaining to a condition caused by treatment, medications, or diagnostic procedures

Lipemic Pertaining to turbidity (serum or plasma appears cloudy white) from increased lipid content in the blood

Petechiae Small red spots appearing on the skin

Preexamination Variable Processes that occur before collection of a sample

Syncope Fainting

INTRODUCTION

Technical and patient complications can occur with blood collection. Technical complications with the venipuncture procedure can result in the inability to obtain blood, a rejected sample, or discomfort to the patient. This chapter identifies the complications that can be encountered and remedies for each. Patient preexamination variables and their effect on laboratory tests also are included.

PREEXAMINATION VARIABLES

Preexamination variables are associated with the patient's activities before sample collection that can affect the quality of the sample. As can be seen in **Table 4-1,** many patient activities can cause variations in a number of laboratory tests. Other than ensuring that a patient with a requisition for fasting tests has not eaten before having blood drawn, there is little that the blood collector can do about those. However, failure to fast can be the cause of a rejected specimen because of **lipemic** serum. Tests on older patients can be affected by posture, and a requisition may request that the patient either lie down or sit down for a specified length of time.

Basal State

After the patient has refrained from strenuous exercise and has not ingested food or beverages except water for 12 hours (known as the **basal state**) is the ideal time to

---

TABLE 4-1 Major Tests Affected by Patient Preexamination Variables

Variable	Increased Results	Decreased Results
Nonfasting	Glucose, triglycerides, aspartate aminotransferase (AST), bilirubin, blood urea nitrogen (BUN), phosphorus, uric acid, growth hormone, cholesterol, lipoproteins (high-density lipoprotein [HDL], low-density lipoprotein [LDL])	
Prolonged fasting	Bilirubin, ketones, lactate, fatty acids, glucagon, and triglycerides	Glucose, insulin, cholesterol, and thyroid hormones
Posture	Albumin, aldosterone, bilirubin, calcium, cortisol, enzymes, cholesterol, total protein, triglycerides, red blood cells (RBCs), white blood cells (WBCs), thyroxine (T_4), plasma renin, serum aldosterone, and catecholamines	
Short-term exercise	Creatinine, fatty acids, lactate, AST, creatine kinase (CK), lactate dehydrogenase (LD), uric acid, bilirubin, HDL, hormones, aldosterone, renin, angiotensin, and WBCs	Arterial pH and P_{CO_2}

TABLE 4-1 **Major Tests Affected by Patient Preexamination Variables—cont'd**

Variable	Increased Results	Decreased Results
Long-term exercise	Aldolase, creatinine, sex hormones, AST, CK, and LD	
Stress	Adrenal hormones, aldosterone, renin, thyroid-stimulating hormone (TSH), growth hormone (GH), prolactin, Po_2, and WBCs	Serum iron and Pco_2
Alcohol	Glucose, aldosterone, prolactin, cortisol, cholesterol, triglycerides, luteinizing hormone (LH), catecholamine, AST, alanine transaminase (ALT), estradiol, mean corpuscular volume (MCV), HDL, and iron	Testosterone
Caffeine	Fatty acids, hormone levels, glycerol, lipoproteins, and serum gastrin	
Smoking	Glucose, BUN, triglycerides, cholesterol, alkaline phosphatase (ALP), catecholamines, cortisol, IgE, hemoglobin, hematocrit, RBCs, and WBCs	Immunoglobulins IgA, IgG, and IgM
Altitude	RBCs, hemoglobin, and hematocrit	
Age	Cholesterol and triglycerides	Hormones
Pregnancy	Protein, ALP, estradiol, free fatty acids, iron, and RBCs	Erythrocyte sedimentation rate (ESR), and factors II, V, VII, IX, X
Dehydration	Calcium, coagulation factors, enzymes, iron, RBCs, and sodium (NA)	
Diurnal variation (a.m.)	Cortisol, testosterone, bilirubin, hemoglobin, insulin, potassium, renin, RBCs, TSH, LH, follicle-stimulating hormone (FSH), estradiol, aldosterone, and serum iron	Eosinophils, creatinine, glucose, phosphate, and triglycerides

Reproduced with permission from Strasinger, S.K., and Di Lorenzo, M.S.: The Phlebotomy Textbook, ed. 3. Philadelphia, F.A. Davis, 2011.

collect blood from a patient. Reference values for laboratory tests are determined from a normal, representative sample of volunteers who are in a basal state.

Diet

The ingestion of food and beverages alters the level of certain blood components. The tests most affected are lipids and glucose. Serum or plasma collected from patients shortly after a meal may appear cloudy or turbid (lipemic) **(Fig. 4-1)** owing to the presence of fatty substances. For most tests, the patient is required to fast for 10 to 12 hours (no food or drink, except water). As shown in **Table 4-1,** prolonged fasting, however, can also alter certain blood tests. When a **fasting** sample is requested, it is the responsibility of the blood collector to determine whether the patient has been fasting for the required length of time. If the patient has not, and the health-care provider still wants the test, it must be noted on the requisition that the sample is "nonfasting."

Posture

Changes in patient posture from a supine to an erect position cause variations in some blood constituents, such as cellular elements, plasma proteins, compounds bound to plasma proteins, and high molecular weight substances. The large size of these substances prevents their movement between the plasma and tissue fluid when body position changes. Therefore, when a person moves from a supine to an erect position and water leaves the plasma, the concentration of these substances increases in the plasma. **Table 4-1** lists the tests most noticeably affected. The concentration of these analytes can increase 4 percent to 15 percent within 10 minutes after changing from a supine position to standing. After returning to the supine position from standing, it takes about 30 minutes for the analytes to decrease to the original level. This is most noticeable in patients with disorders such as congestive heart failure and liver disease that cause increased fluid to remain in the tissue.

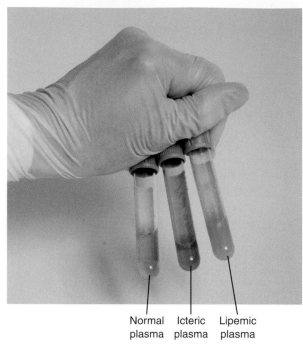

Normal   Icteric   Lipemic
plasma   plasma   plasma

FIGURE 4-1 Normal, icteric, and lipemic specimens. *(Reproduced with permission from Strasinger, S.K., and Di Lorenzo, M.S.: The Phlebotomy Textbook, ed. 3. Philadelphia, F.A. Davis, 2011.)*

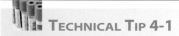 **TECHNICAL TIP 4-1**

Asking elderly patients to sit while you are checking their identification and arranging the equipment can allow the patient's blood to stabilize.

Exercise

Moderate or strenuous exercise affects laboratory test results, as shown in **Table 4-1.** The effects of exercise depend on the physical fitness and muscle mass of the patient, the strenuousness and intensity of the exercise, and the time between the exercise and blood collection. The values usually return to normal within several hours of relaxation in a healthy person; however, skeletal muscles may be elevated for 24 hours.

Stress

Failure to calm a frightened, nervous patient before sample collection may increase levels of certain analytes, as listed in **Table 4-1.** It has been reported that white blood cell (WBC) counts collected from a crying baby may be markedly elevated. In contrast, WBC counts in early morning samples collected from patients in a basal state will be decreased until normal activity is resumed. Elevated WBC counts return to normal within 1 hour.

 TECHNICAL TIP 4-2

For an accurate WBC count, discontinue blood collection from a crying child until after the child has been calm for at least 1 hour.

Smoking

The effects of smoking on laboratory test results are shown in **Table 4-1.** The extent of the effect depends on the type and the number of cigarettes smoked and the amount of smoke inhaled.

Smoking affects the levels of immunoglobulins, lowering the effectiveness of the immune system. Because of the risk of infection, surgery may be postponed.

Altitude

Red blood cell (RBC) counts and hemoglobin and hematocrit values are increased in high-altitude areas such as the mountains where there are reduced oxygen levels. Reference ranges for RBC parameters must be established for populations living higher than 5,000 feet above sea level.

Age and Gender

Laboratory results vary in infancy, childhood, adulthood, and the elderly because of the gradual change in the composition of body fluids. Reference ranges are established for the different patient age and gender groups; therefore, the age or date of birth and gender of the patient must be present on the requisition form.

Pregnancy

Pregnancy-related differences in laboratory test results are caused by physiological changes in the body including increases in plasma volume. The increased plasma volume may cause a dilutional effect and lower certain analytes, as listed in **Table 4-1.**

Diurnal Variation

The concentration of some blood constituents is affected by the time of day. Diurnal rhythm is the normal fluctuation in blood levels at different times of the day based on a 24-hour cycle of eating and sleeping. Blood analytes are released into the bloodstream intermittently. **Table 4-1** lists the major analytes affected by **diurnal variation.**

TECHNICAL TIP 4-3

Cortisol and iron levels can differ by 50 percent between 8 a.m. and 4 p.m.; therefore, it is important to collect samples for analytes that exhibit diurnal variation at the correct scheduled time.

Medications

Certain medications **(Table 4-2)** may affect a patient's test results, either by changing a metabolic process within the patient or by producing interference with the testing procedure. IV administration of dyes used in diagnostic procedures also can interfere with testing procedures. Fortunately, the patient's health-care provider will know about these.

TECHNICAL TIP 4-4

Patients taking blood thinners will usually mention this; however, it is a good practice to ask the patient whether he or she is taking a blood thinner, indicating that additional pressure may be needed after collection.

TECHNICAL COMPLICATIONS

Failure to Obtain Blood

The primary complication for the blood collector is the failure to obtain blood when the needle is inserted. **Figure 4-2** illustrates possible causes of failure to obtain blood. Slightly moving or turning the needle may result in blood flow without having to repuncture the patient.

Needle Beside the Vein

A frequent reason for the failure to obtain blood occurs when a vein is not well anchored prior to the puncture. The needle may slip to the side of the vein without actual penetration ("rolling vein") **(see Fig 4-2H).** Gently touching the area around the needle with a cleansed, gloved finger may determine the positions of

---

TABLE 4-2 **Common Medications Affecting Laboratory Tests**	
Medication	**Affected Tests/Systems**
Acetaminophen and certain antibiotics	Elevated liver enzymes and bilirubin
Cholesterol-lowering drugs	Prolonged PT and APTT
Certain antibiotics	Elevated BUN, creatinine, and electrolyte imbalance
Corticosteroids and estrogen diuretics	Elevated amylase and lipase
Diuretics	Increased calcium, glucose, and uric acid and decreased sodium and potassium
Chemotherapy	Decreased RBCs, WBCs, and platelets
Aspirin, salicylates, and herbal supplements	Prolonged PT and bleeding time
Radiographic contrast media	Routine urinalysis
Fluorescein dye	Increased creatinine, cortisol, and digoxin
Oral contraceptives	Decreased apoproteins, transcortin, cholesterol, HDL, triglycerides, LH, FSH, ferritin, and iron

APTT = activated partial thromboplastin time; BUN = blood urea nitrogen; FSH = follicle stimulating hormone; HDL = high-density lipoprotein; LH = luteinizing hormone; PT = prothrombin time; RBCs = red blood cells; WBCs = white blood cells.

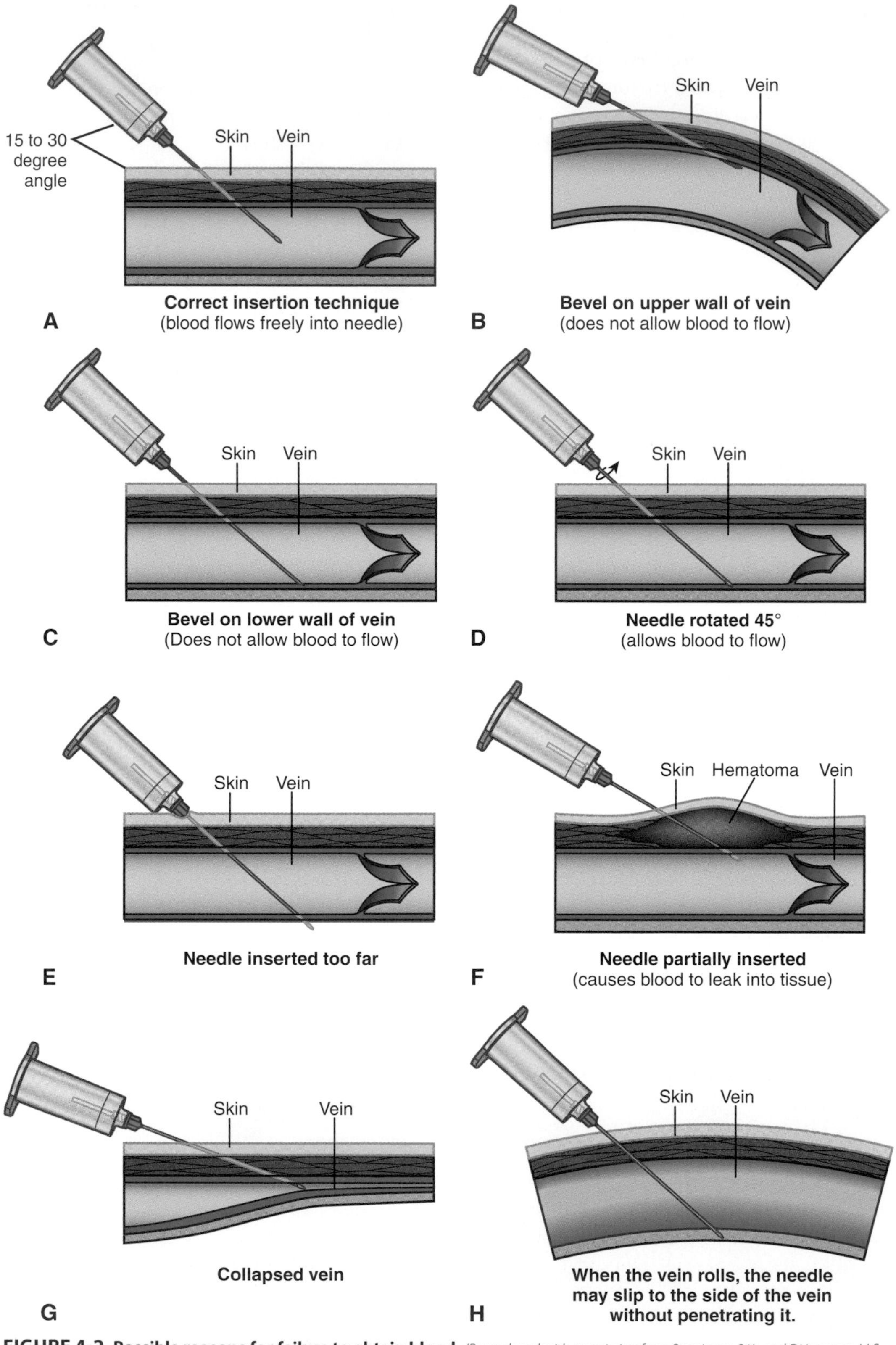

FIGURE 4-2 Possible reasons for failure to obtain blood. *(Reproduced with permission from Strasinger, S.K., and Di Lorenzo, M.S.: The Phlebotomy Textbook, ed. 3. Philadelphia, F.A. Davis, 2011.)*

the vein and the needle, and allow the needle to be slightly redirected. To avoid having to repuncture the patient, withdraw the needle until the bevel is just under the skin, reanchor the vein, and redirect the needle into the vein.

Needle Too Deep

Blood flow may not occur when the angle of needle insertion is too steep (greater than 30 degrees) or when the tube holder is not kept steady when tubes are advanced on to the needle. The needle may penetrate through the vein into the tissue. Gently pulling the needle back may produce blood flow **(see Fig. 4-2E).**

Needle Too Shallow

If the needle angle is too shallow (less than 15 degrees), the needle may only partially enter the lumen of the vein, causing blood to leak into the tissues. Slowly advancing the needle into the vein may correct the problem **(see Fig. 4-2F).**

Bevel Against the Wall of the Vein

Blood flow also may be prevented when the bevel of the needle is resting against the upper or lower wall of the vein. Pulling slightly back on the needle will allow blood to flow freely **(see Fig. 4-2, B, C, and D).**

Collapsed Vein

Using too large an evacuated tube or pulling back on the plunger of a syringe too quickly creates suction pressure that can cause a vein to collapse and stop blood flow **(see Fig. 4-2G).** Using a smaller evacuated tube or pulling more slowly on the syringe plunger may remedy the situation. If this does not help, another puncture must be performed, possibly using a syringe or a winged blood collection set.

Faulty Evacuated Tube

If the needle appears to be in the vein and there is no blood flow to the tube, a faulty tube may be the problem. Loss of vacuum in an evacuated tube can be caused by manufacturer error, age of the tube, dropping the tube, or accidental puncture when assembling the equipment. A new tube should be used. A tube can be used only once.

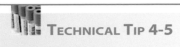

TECHNICAL TIP 4-5

Remember to always have extra tubes within reach.

It is important for blood collectors to know these techniques to avoid having the patient unnecessarily repunctured. Movement of the needle should not include blind or vigorous probing, because not only is this painful to the patient, but this also enlarges the puncture site and blood may leak into the tissues and form a hematoma. The most critical permanent injury in the venipuncture procedure caused by vigorous probing is damage to the median antebrachial cutaneous nerve. Errors in technique that cause injury include selecting high-risk venipuncture sites, employing an excessive angle of needle insertion, and excessive manipulation of the needle.

SAFETY TIP 4-1

CLSI standard GP41-A6 (H3-A6) limits needle redirection only to a forward or backward movement in a straight line.

TECHNICAL TIP 4-6

Probing and lateral movements of the needle particularly near the basilic vein are the main causes of accidental arterial punctures and nerve injury.

Collection Attempts

When blood is not obtained from the initial venipuncture, the blood collector should select another site, either in the other arm or below the previous site, **and repeat the procedure using a new needle.** If the second puncture is not successful, the same person should not make another attempt. Another qualified person in your facility or a phlebotomist from the clinical laboratory should attempt to collect the sample.

HEMATOMAS

Hematomas are caused by the leakage of blood into the tissues around the venipuncture site. The skin discoloration and swelling that accompany a hematoma are often a cause of anxiety and discomfort to the patient, and can cause disabling compression injury to nerves **(Fig. 4-3).** Improper technique when removing the needle is a frequent cause of the appearance of a hematoma on the patient's arm.

Errors in technique that cause blood to leak or to be forced into the surrounding tissue and produce hematomas include the following:

1. Failing to remove the tourniquet prior to removing the needle
2. Applying inadequate pressure to the site after removal of the needle

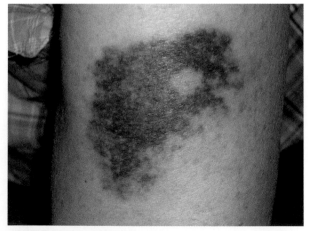

FIGURE 4-3 Hematoma formed from venipuncture. *(Reproduced with permission from Strasinger, S.K., and Di Lorenzo, M.S.: The Phlebotomy Textbook, ed. 3. Philadelphia, F.A. Davis, 2011.)*

3. Excessive probing to obtain blood
4. Failing to insert the needle far enough into the vein
5. Inserting the needle through the vein
6. Bending the arm while applying pressure
7. Using veins that are fragile or too small for the needle size
8. Selecting a needle too large for the vein
9. Accidentally puncturing the brachial artery

Under normal conditions, the elasticity of the vein walls prevents the leakage of blood around the needle during venipuncture. A decrease in the elasticity of the vein walls in geriatric patients causes them to be more prone to developing hematomas. If the area begins to form a hematoma while blood is being collected, immediately remove the tourniquet and needle and apply pressure to the site for 2 minutes. Using small-bore needles and firmly anchoring the veins prior to needle insertion may prevent hematoma formation in these patients. A cold compress may be offered to the patient to minimize hematoma swelling and pain. Follow facility policy.

The compromised venipuncture site is unacceptable for blood collection until the hematoma is resolved. An alternative site should be chosen for venipuncture, or if none is available, the venipuncture must be performed below the hematoma. The goal of successful blood collection is not only to obtain the sample, but also to preserve the site for future venipunctures. It is critical to prevent hematoma formation.

Compartment Syndrome

Some patients receiving anticoagulants or who have a coagulation disorder (hemophilia) may continue to bleed large amounts of blood into the subcutaneous tissue surrounding the puncture site. The blood can accumulate within the tissues of the muscles that surround the arm or hand and cause an increased pressure to build in the area, which can interfere with blood flow and cause muscle injury. This condition called, **compartment syndrome,** can cause pain, swelling, numbness, and permanent injury to the nerves. This is a serious condition and would require a surgical procedure to open the compartment to relieve the pressure. This syndrome can be prevented by checking the venipuncture site for bleeding and hematoma formation before applying the bandage.

NERVE INJURY

Temporary or permanent nerve damage can be caused by incorrect vein site selection or improper venipuncture technique and may result in loss of movement to the arm or hand, and the possibility of a lawsuit. Symptoms of nerve involvement are tingling, a burning or electric shock sensation, pain that is felt up and down the arm, or a numbness of the arm. The factors associated with nerve injury in blood collection are preventable and include the following:

- Improper vein selection (underside of the wrist, basilic vein)
- Using jerky movements
- Inserting the needle too far (inserting the needle at greater than 30-degree angle)
- Movement by the patient while the needle is in the vein
- Lateral redirection of the needle
- Blind probing

IATROGENIC ANEMIA

Iatrogenic anemia pertains to a condition of blood loss caused by treatment. This is especially dangerous for infants and the geriatric population. Removal of more than 10 percent of a patient's blood can be life threatening in these patients. Collecting the minimum amount of blood, monitoring collection orders for duplicate requests, and avoiding redraws can reduce excessive blood collections.

HEMOLYZED SAMPLES

The most common cause of preexamination error is **hemolysis.** It is detected by the presence of pink or red plasma or serum **(Fig. 4-4).** Rupture of the red blood cell membrane releases cellular contents into the serum or plasma that produces interference with many test results, which may require the sample to be recollected. **Table 4-3** summarizes the major tests affected by hemolysis.

Errors in performance of the venipuncture account for the majority of hemolyzed samples and include the following:

1. Using a needle of too small a diameter (above 23 gauge)
2. Using a small needle with a large evacuated tube
3. Using an improperly attached needle on a syringe so that frothing occurs as the blood enters the syringe
4. Pulling the plunger of a syringe back too fast
5. Drawing blood from a site containing a hematoma

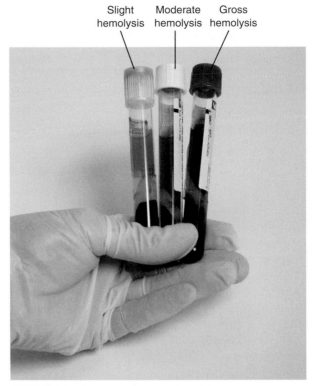

FIGURE 4-4 **Slight, moderate, and gross hemolysis.** *(Reproduced with permission from Strasinger, S.K., and Di Lorenzo, M.S.: The Phlebotomy Textbook, ed. 3. Philadelphia, F.A. Davis, 2011.)*

6. Vigorously mixing tubes
7. Forcing blood from a syringe into an evacuated tube
8. Collecting samples from IV lines when not recommended by the manufacturer
9. Applying the tourniquet too close to the puncture site or for too long a time period
10. Using fragile hand veins
11. Performing venipuncture before the alcohol is allowed to dry
12. Collecting blood through different internal diameters of catheters and connectors
13. Partially filling sodium fluoride tubes
14. Readjusting the needle in the vein or using occluded veins

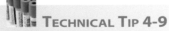 **TECHNICAL TIP 4-9**

Hemolysis that is not evident to the naked eye can elevate critical potassium values.

TABLE 4-3 Laboratory Tests Affected by Hemolysis

Seriously Affected	Noticeably Affected	Slightly Affected
Potassium (K)	Serum iron (Fe)	Phosphorus (P)
Lactic dehydrogenase (LD)	Alanine aminotransferase (ALT)	Total protein (TP)
Aspartate aminotransferase (AST)	Thyroxine (T_4)	Albumin
Complete blood count (CBC)	Prothrombin time (PT)	Magnesium (Mg)
	Activated partial thromboplastin (APTT)	Calcium (Ca)
	C-peptide	Alkaline phosphatase (ALP)
		Rapid plasma reagin (RPR)

 TECHNICAL TIP 4-10

Potassium values are higher in serum than in plasma because of the release of potassium from platelets during clotting.

Factors in processing, handling, or transporting the sample can result in hemolyzed samples and include the following:

1. Rimming clots
2. Prolonged contact of serum or plasma with cells
3. Centrifuging at a higher than recommended speed and with increased heat exposure in the centrifuge
4. Elevated or decreased temperatures of blood
5. Using pneumatic tube systems or transport containers without shock-absorbing padding

Various patient physiological factors affect hemolysis and include the following:

1. Metabolic disorders (liver disease, sickle cell anemia, autoimmune hemolytic anemia, blood transfusion reactions)
2. Chemical agents (lead, sulfonamides, antimalarial drugs, analgesics)
3. Physical agents (mechanical heart valve, third-degree burns)
4. Infectious agents (parasites, bacteria)

SAMPLE CONTAMINATION

Sample contamination affects the integrity of the sample, causing invalid test results. The laboratory personnel may not know that contamination has occurred and consequently might report erroneous test results that adversely affect overall patient care. Incorrect blood collection techniques that cause contamination include the following:

1. Blood collected from edematous areas
2. Blood collected from veins with hematomas
3. Blood collected from arms containing an IV
4. Sites contaminated with alcohol or iodine
5. Anticoagulant carryover between tubes

TUBE PROBLEMS

Rarely, the blood collector may encounter an evacuated tube that pops back or off the back of the holder needle while blood is being collected. Readvancing the tube onto the needle in the holder and holding it in this position until the tube is filled will remedy this situation.

When using the evacuated tube system, always screw the needle onto the holder tightly. Needles can become unscrewed from the holder during venipuncture. If this happens, release the tourniquet immediately, and carefully remove the needle. Activate the safety device over the needle.

Reflux of a tube anticoagulant can occur when there is blood backflow into a patient's vein from the collection tube. This can cause adverse reactions in the patient. Keeping the patient's arm and the tube in a downward position, allowing the collection tubes to fill from the bottom up, eliminates this problem.

Partially filled collection tubes deliver the wrong ratio of blood to anticoagulant, resulting in an inadequate sample for laboratory testing. Examples of an incorrect ratio of blood to anticoagulant can result in the following:

- Excess liquid anticoagulant in light blue stopper tubes dilutes the plasma and causes prolonged coagulation results.
- Excess ethylenediaminetetraacetic acid (EDTA) in the lavender stopper tube shrinks the red blood cells and affects the hematocrit, red blood cell count, hemoglobin, red blood cell indices, and erythrocyte sedimentation rate (ESR) results.
- Completely filled green stopper tubes are critical for ionized calcium tests.
- Underfilled gray stopper tubes cause hemolysis of the red blood cells.

Serum separator tubes (SSTs) and red stopper tubes are usually not affected by partially filled collection tubes providing there is an adequate amount of sample to perform the test. "Partial-draw" tubes are available for situations in which it is difficult to obtain a full tube. These tubes have a smaller amount of vacuum. A line is present on each tube to indicate the proper fill level.

TECHNICAL TIP 4-11

To ensure prevention of reflux, blood in the tubes should not come in contact with the stopper during collection.

PATIENT COMPLICATIONS

Fainting (Syncope)

Apprehensive patients may be prone to fainting (**syncope**). It is sometimes possible to detect such patients during vein palpation, because their skin may feel cold and clammy. Other signs include pallor, perspiration, or the patient indicating that he or she feels light-headed, dizzy, or nauseous.

The blood collector should ask the patient whether he or she had previous problems with blood collection or a tendency to faint. Having the patient lie down or using a blood collection chair with a locked armrest will prevent the patient from falling and injuring him- or herself. Distracting the patient through conversation may be helpful.

If a patient begins to faint during the procedure, remove the tourniquet and needle and apply pressure to the venipuncture site. Make certain a patient who is not in bed is supported and that the patient lowers his or her head. Applying cold compresses to the forehead and back of the neck helps revive the patient. Outpatients who have been fasting for prolonged periods should be given something sweet to drink and be required to remain in the area for 15 to 30 minutes. All incidents of syncope should be documented according to facility policy.

TECHNICAL TIP 4-12

According to CLSI standard GP41-A6 (H3-A6), the use of ammonia inhalants for a fainting patient is not advised.

Seizures

It is rare for patients to develop seizures during venipuncture. If this happens, the needle and tourniquet should be removed, pressure applied to the site, and help summoned. Restrain the patient only to the extent that injury is prevented. Do not attempt to place anything in the patient's mouth. Document the time the seizure started and stopped according to facility policy.

TECHNICAL TIP 4-13

Patients frequently mention previous adverse reactions. If these patients are sitting up, it may be wise to have them lie down prior to collection. It is not uncommon for patients with a history of fainting to faint again.

Petechiae

Patients who present with small, nonraised red hemorrhagic spots (called petechiae) may have prolonged bleeding following venipuncture. **Petechiae** can be an indication of a coagulation disorder, such as a low platelet count or abnormal platelet function. Be sure to apply additional pressure to the site until the bleeding stops.

Allergies

Patients are occasionally allergic to alcohol, iodine, latex, or the glue used in adhesive bandages. Necessary precautions must be observed by using alternative antiseptics, paper tape, or self-adhering wrap and nonlatex products.

SPECIAL PATIENT POPULATIONS

Unique preparation and sometimes modifications to the blood collection technique are necessary to successfully accommodate the collection of blood from the pediatric and geriatric populations.

Geriatric Population

Blood collection in the geriatric population presents a challenge to the blood collector. Physical, emotional, and physiological factors related to the aging process can cause difficulty with the blood collection procedure and sample integrity. Patients often are embarrassed by these conditions, which may cause anxiety or fear of blood collection. The goal is to perform a nontraumatic venipuncture without bruising or excessive bleeding and provide a quality sample for analysis.

Physical Factors

Physical changes that occur in the geriatric patient that have an effect on blood collection include the following:

- Normal aging often results in gradual hearing loss. The blood collector must face the patient and speak clearly and repeat instructions if necessary. Use of nonverbal methods or paper and pencil to explain the procedure and obtain permission may be required before blood collection.
- Failing eyesight is common in the geriatric patient. The patient may have to be guided to the blood drawing chair and have help being seated.
- Muscle weakness may cause the patient to be unable to make a fist before venipuncture or to hold the gauze after the venipuncture.
- Memory loss may cause the geriatric patient not to remember medications he or she may have taken that can affect laboratory test results. A patient's inability to remember when he or she has last eaten can affect a test requiring fasting.
- Malnutrition or dehydration because of not eating or drinking adequately can make locating veins for venipuncture difficult because of decreased plasma volume and can affect laboratory results by raising potassium levels.

Disease States

Certain disease states found predominantly in the geriatric population contribute to the challenge of venipuncture and include the following:

- A patient with Alzheimer's disease may be confused or combative, which can cause problems with identification and performing the procedure. Assistance from a family member or the patient's caretaker is often necessary to calm the patient and hold the arm steady.
- Stroke patients may have paralysis or speech impairments that require assistance in positioning and holding the arm and help with communication.
- Arthritic patients may be in pain or unable to straighten the arm and may require assistance gently positioning and holding the arm. Using a winged blood collection set with flexible tubing will allow the blood collector to access veins at awkward angles.
- Geriatric patients are often on anticoagulant therapy for heart problems or stroke. Extra time is necessary to hold pressure on the site until bleeding has stopped before bandaging the area to avoid excessive bleeding or hematoma formation.
- Geriatric patients may have tremors, as evidenced in Parkinson disease, and cannot hold the arm still for the venipuncture procedure.

Physiological Changes

The following physiological changes in the aging process affect venipuncture:

- Epidermal cell replacement in the aging patient is delayed, increasing the chance of infection. If the patient already has a weakened immune system, the patient may not heal as quickly or have the ability to fight bacteria that can be introduced during venipuncture. Extra care must be taken when preparing the site for venipuncture.
- The loss of collagen and subcutaneous tissue makes the veins less elastic and fragile with a tendency to collapse. The veins are harder to anchor and puncture and more prone to hematoma formation. The blood collector must firmly anchor the vein below the site so that the vein does not move when it is punctured. Loose skin can be pulled taut by wrapping your hand

around the arm from behind. The angle of the needle may need to be decreased for venipuncture because the veins are often close to the surface.

- Arteries and veins often become sclerotic in the older patient, making them poor sites for venipuncture because of the compromised blood flow.

Site Selection

The antecubital fossa may not be the best site for venipuncture in the geriatric patient because of the difficulty in locating and anchoring veins. Often hematomas from previous venipunctures are present and render the site unusable for blood collection. Techniques previously described such as warming the site can make the vein more prominent. Never tap the vein to avoid bruising the patient. The veins in the hand or forearm may be a better choice.

Equipment Selection

The evacuated tube system (ETS) is usually not the best choice for venipuncture on the geriatric patient because the vacuum pressure in the collection tube may cause fragile veins to collapse. A better choice is a winged blood collection set with a 23-gauge needle attached to a syringe that will allow the blood collector to control the suction pressure on the vein. A small gauge needle with a syringe is also an option. Partial-draw tubes should be used because of the tendency to develop anemia by geriatric patients; therefore, the volume of blood collected should be kept to the minimum acceptable amount.

Tourniquet and Bandage Application

Blood pressure cuffs can be used for the thin patient with small, hard-to-find veins. Geriatric patients are prone to bruising when the tourniquet or adhesive bandages are applied. Injury can be avoided by placing a tourniquet over the patient's sleeve. Self-adhering bandages are a preferable choice for the geriatric patient. Adhesive bandages on the fragile skin of geriatric patients can take off a layer of skin when they are removed. This can leave a raw wound that is susceptible to infection. A better alternative is for the blood collector to hold pressure on the site for 3 to 5 minutes or until the bleeding has stopped.

Additional Considerations

Dermal puncture, when possible, should be performed on the geriatric patient as a way of avoiding complications,

such as hematomas, bruising, collapsed veins, and anemia. The advances in point-of-care testing have made it possible to perform many types of tests on a small amount of blood that can be obtained by dermal puncture.

Pediatric Population

Ideally, children younger than 2 years of age should have blood collected by dermal puncture procedure (see Chapter 6). However, special tests for coagulation, erythrocyte sedimentation rates, special diagnostic studies, or blood cultures require more blood than can be collected from a finger or heel puncture and must be collected by venipuncture.

Patient/Parent Preparation

Pediatric blood collection involves preparing both the child and parent, using certain restraining procedures and special equipment. Pediatric phlebotomy presents emotional as well as technical difficulties and should be performed only by experienced blood collectors. It is important to keep the patient as calm as possible during the procedure because emotional stress and crying can affect blood analytes and cause erroneous test results. The minimum amount of blood required should be collected for testing because infants and children have smaller blood volumes.

Restraints

Assistance is usually required when collecting blood from a small child. Physical restraint may be required to immobilize the young child and steady the arm for the venipuncture procedure. This can be accomplished by having someone hold the child in either a vertical or horizontal restraint. In the vertical position, the parent holds the child in an upright position on the lap. The parent places an arm around the toddler to hold the arm not being used. Using the other arm, the parent holds the child's venipuncture arm firmly from behind, at the bend of the elbow, in a downward position.

In the horizontal restraint, the child lies down, with the parent on one side of the bed and the blood collector on the opposite side. The parent leans over the child holding the near arm and body securely while reaching over the body to hold the opposite venipuncture arm for the blood collector.

Equipment Selection

The minimum amount of blood required for laboratory testing should be collected from infants and small children because drawing excessive amounts of blood can cause anemia. The amount of blood collected within a 24-hour period must be monitored because of the small blood volume in newborns and small children. When using an ETS, select the smallest evacuated tube available, allowing for collection of the least amount of blood and protecting the vein from collapse. Evacuated tubes as small as 1.8 mL are available. A 23-gauge winged blood collection set needle with a syringe is recommended because of the small, fragile veins. If only a very small amount of blood is collected, use a microcollection tube rather than an evacuated tube. Pediatric-sized tourniquets also are available.

Pain Interventions

A local topical anesthetic, eutectic mixture of local anesthetics (EMLA) is ideal for use on an apprehensive child before venipuncture. This emulsion of lidocaine and prilocaine is applied directly to intact skin and covered with an occlusive dressing. EMLA penetrates to a depth of 5 mm through the epidermal and dermal layers of the skin. It takes 60 minutes to reach its optimal effect and lasts for 2 or 3 hours. EMLA should not be used on infants younger than 1 month of age or if the child is allergic to local anesthetics. One side effect of this emulsion may be pallor at the site or a slight redness because of the adhesive covering. Numbing sprays that have an immediate effect are also available.

It has been shown that a sucrose solution has a calming effect on infants. Commercial sucrose pacifiers or nipples are available. A 24 percent solution of sucrose may be made by mixing 4 teaspoons of water with 1 teaspoon of sugar. This sucrose solution may be given to the infant using a syringe, dropper, nipple, or pacifier about 2 minutes before venipuncture, and the effects last for about 5 minutes.

Site Selection

The veins located in the antecubital fossa or the forearms are the best choice for children older than 2 years of age. Do not use deep veins.

CAUSES OF SAMPLE REJECTION

Samples brought to the laboratory may be rejected if conditions are present that would compromise the validity of the test results. Rejection of a sample has clinical consequences because it delays making laboratory results available for the health-care provider, delays patient treatment, and causes inconvenience and discomfort for the patient.

Major reasons for sample rejection include the following:

1. Unlabeled or mislabeled samples
2. Inadequate volume
3. Collection in the wrong tube
4. Hemolysis
5. Lipemia
6. Clotted blood in an anticoagulant tube
7. Improper handling during transport, such as not chilling the sample
8. Samples without a requisition form
9. Contaminated sample containers
10. Delays in processing the sample
11. Use of outdated blood collection tubes

BIBLIOGRAPHY

CLSI: *Procedures for the Collection of Diagnostic Blood Specimens by Venipuncture*, ed. 6. Approved Guideline GP41-A6 (H03-A6). Wayne, PA, CLSI, 2007.

CLSI: *Procedures for the Handling and Processing of Blood Specimens for Common Laboratory Tests*, ed. 4. Approved Guideline GP44-A4 (H18-A4). Wayne, PA, CLSI, 2012.

Strasinger, S.K., and DiLorenzo, M.S.: *The Phlebotomy Textbook*, ed. 3. Philadelphia, PA, F.A. Davis, 2011.

INTERNET RESOURCES

www.clsi.org

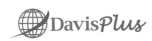 For additional material, please visit http://davisplus.fadavis.com.

REVIEW QUESTIONS

1. Which of the following techniques are acceptable when blood is not obtained after needle insertion?
   a. Gently advancing the needle
   b. Gently pulling the needle back
   c. Inserting a new tube into the holder
   d. All of the above

2. Which of the following is most critically affected in a hemolyzed specimen?
   a. Potassium
   b. Albumin
   c. Total protein
   d. Calcium

3. What should the blood collector do first when a patient develops syncope?
   a. Lower the patient's head
   b. Apply cold compresses to the patient's neck
   c. Remove the tourniquet and needle
   d. Place the patient on a bed

4. When performing venipuncture on a pediatric patient, the blood collector may require:
   a. Assistance
   b. A pediatric requisition
   c. Partial-draw evacuated tubes
   d. Both a and c

5. Geriatric patients are more prone to hematoma formation because:
   a. They have smaller veins
   b. Tourniquets must be tied tighter
   c. Their veins have decreased elasticity
   d. They have difficulty making a fist

6. Which of the following reasons would cause a sample to be rejected?
   a. Clots in a lavender stopper tube
   b. Collection in a partial-draw tube
   c. Incompletely filled SST tube
   d. Clots in a red stopper tube

7. What can cause blood to begin to flow and then stop after the evacuated tube is pushed onto the needle?
   a. An occluded vein
   b. Collapsing of the vein
   c. The bevel of the needle resting on the vein wall
   d. All of the above

8. A patient is scheduled to have a blood sample drawn at 0800 and again at 1600. The reason for these instructions is that:
   a. The patient will be fasting for the 0800 sample.
   b. The patient will be more stressed after just waking up
   c. The substance being tested exhibits diurnal variation
   d. The laboratory may be too busy to analyze the 0800 sample on time.

9. Which of the following can cause hematoma formation?
   a. Inserting the needle through the vein
   b. Bending the arm while applying pressure
   c. Excessive probing
   d. All of the above

10. Match the following patient variables with the possible effect on test results:
    a. _____ Decreased glucose   1. Stress
    b. _____ Increased hemoglobin   2. Long-term exercise
    c. _____ Increased white blood cells   3. Prolonged fasting
    d. _____ Increased creatine kinase   4. Altitude

FOR FURTHER STUDY

1. How should you proceed after no blood has been obtained from a patient's left antecubital area and blood stops flowing from the right antecubital before the sample collection is complete?
2. What is a possible reason for the stoppage of blood flow during a sample collection after a successful puncture is performed, and what are two methods by which the required blood can be collected?
3. What are possible causes for swelling at a puncture site when collecting a sample using routine evacuated tube equipment, and how can the sample be collected?

CASE STUDY 4-1

Tom, an extremely overweight man, came to the physician's office laboratory with a requisition form for a metabolic profile. Mary, the blood collector, had a difficult time finding a good median cubital or cephalic vein; however, she did feel a deep basilic vein. Inserting the needle at a greater than 30-degree angle and after much probing, Mary was able to obtain the blood. Tom complained of a burning, tingling sensation up and down his arm.

1. What caused the tingling sensation?
2. What is the CLSI recommendation for needle angle and vein selection?
3. What other complication may have occurred that would cause the laboratory to reject the sample?

CASE STUDY 4-2

While blood for a CBC is being collected, Kathy, the patient, develops syncope. Marcia, the blood collector, removes the needle and lowers Kathy's head. Once Kathy has recovered, Marcia labels the lavender stopper tube, which contains enough blood, and delivers it to the clinical laboratory. Many results from this sample are markedly lower than those from Kathy's previous CBC.

1. How could the quality of the sample have caused this discrepancy?
2. How could the venipuncture complication have contributed to this error?
3. Could Marcia have done anything differently? Explain your answer.

Special Blood Collection

LEARNING OBJECTIVES

Upon completion of this chapter, the reader will be able to:

5.1 Define the various test collection priorities.

5.2 Explain the requirements for oral glucose tolerance tests (OGTTs).

5.3 Discuss diurnal variation of blood constituents and list three substances that would be affected.

5.4 Differentiate between a trough and a peak level in therapeutic drug monitoring and state the importance for collecting the sample at the prescribed time.

5.5 Discuss the timing sequences for the collection of blood cultures, the reasons for selecting a particular timing sequence, and the number of samples collected.

5.6 Describe the equipment, procedure, and precautions associated with arterial puncture.

5.7 Explain the effects of sample handling and transport on test results.

5.8 Describe the procedure for collecting samples for cold agglutinins and cryoglobulins.

5.9 List eight tests for which samples must be chilled immediately after collection.

5.10 List five tests for which the results are affected by exposure of the sample to light.

5.11 Define chain of custody and state three tests that may require it.

KEY TERMS

Arteriospasm Spontaneous constriction of an artery

Aseptic Free of contamination by microorganisms

Chain of Custody Documentation of the collection and handling of forensic samples

Diurnal Variation Normal changes in blood constituent levels at different times of the day

Peak Level Sample collected when a serum drug level is highest

Septicemia The presence of pathogenic microorganisms in the blood

Steady State A 20- to 30-minute period of controlled stable oxygen consumption and no physical exercise

Trough Level Sample collected when a serum drug level is lowest

Turnaround Time Amount of time between the request for a test and the reporting of results

INTRODUCTION

Certain laboratory tests require the use of techniques that are not part of the routine venipuncture procedure. These procedures may involve patient preparation, timing of sample collection, blood collection techniques, sample handling, and sample transport. The blood collector must know when these techniques are required, how to perform them, and how sample integrity is affected when they are not performed correctly.

COLLECTION PRIORITIES

Test orders are designated as routine, STAT, or timed. **Turnaround times** (TATs) are based on these designations. Routine tests are ordered by the health-care provider to diagnose and monitor a patient's condition. STAT tests have the highest priority. Timed tests must be collected at a specific time. The samples must be delivered to the laboratory promptly and the laboratory personnel notified.

FASTING SAMPLES

Assessment of patient preparation is necessary before blood collection for laboratory tests that require the patient to be fasting or in a basal state. Fasting differs from a basal state condition in that the patient must only have refrained from eating and drinking (except water) for 12 hours, whereas in the basal state the patient also must have refrained from exercise. It is the responsibility of the blood collector to verify that the patient is in the fasting or basal state when required.

 TECHNICAL TIP 5-1

Drinking water is encouraged to avoid dehydration in the patient, which can affect laboratory results.

 TECHNICAL TIP 5-2

A specimen that appears lipemic is an indication that the patient was not fasting and the lipemia may interfere with laboratory testing.

Test results most critically affected in a nonfasting patient are those for glucose, cholesterol, triglycerides, or lipid profiles. If the patient has not fasted, it must be noted on the requisition form. Prolonged fasting increases bilirubin and triglyceride results and markedly decreases glucose levels.

TIMED SAMPLES

Blood collections are frequently requested for specific times, and the timing of sample collection must be strictly followed for accurate test results. Reasons for timed samples are shown in **Box 5-1.**

Collecting a sample early could yield a falsely elevated result, whereas collecting the sample late could yield a falsely normal result. Misinterpretation of test results can cause improper treatment for the patient. The most frequently encountered timed samples are discussed in this chapter.

| BOX 5-1 | **Reasons for Timed Samples** |

Measuring the body's ability to metabolize a particular substance

Monitoring changes in a patient's condition

Determining levels of medications in the blood

Measuring substances that exhibit diurnal variation

Measuring cardiac markers following acute myocardial infarction

Monitoring anticoagulant therapy

Glucose Tolerance Tests

A variety of methods have been available for the diagnosis of diabetes mellitus and gestational diabetes. Originally, these included the 2-hour (hr) postprandial (pp) glucose test and the classic glucose tolerance test (GTT). The 2-hour pp glucose compared a patient's fasting glucose level with the glucose level 2 hours after eating a meal with a high carbohydrate content. The classic GTT required patients to drink a standard glucose load and return for testing on an hourly basis up to 6 hours in length (see Table 5-1 in Procedure 5-1).

The American Diabetes Association (ADA) and the World Health Organization (WHO) have standardized and revised the methods used for the diagnosis of diabetes. Current diagnostic tests for diabetes include an $HgbA_{1C}$ level equal to or greater than 6.5 percent or a fasting plasma glucose equal to or greater than 126 mg/dL or a 2-hr plasma glucose equal to or greater than 200 mg/dL after a 75-g oral glucose tolerance test (OGTT). Gestational diabetes mellitus is diagnosed with the 1-step and 2-step OGTT. The basic instructions for these procedures are similar and are shown in **Procedure 5-1**.

PROCEDURE 5-1 GTT Procedure

EQUIPMENT:

Requisition form	Evacuated tubes
Flavored glucose solution	2×2 gauze
Gloves	Sharps container
Tourniquet	Indelible pen
Alcohol pads	Bandage
Evacuated tube holder and needles	Biohazard bag

PROCEDURE:

Step 1. Identify the patient using normal protocol, explain the procedure, and obtain consent.

Step 2. Confirm that the patient has fasted for 12 hours and not more than 16 hours.

Step 3. Draw a fasting glucose sample. The fasting blood sample is tested before continuing the procedure to determine whether the patient can safely be given a large amount of glucose.

Step 4. Ask the patient to drink the appropriate flavored glucose solution within 5 minutes. Small adults and children may have adjusted amounts based on 1 g of glucose per kilogram of weight.

Oral glucose loads may vary when testing for gestational diabetes.

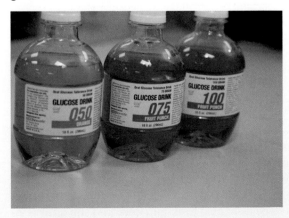

PROCEDURE 5-1 GTT Procedure (Continued)

Step 5. Timing for the remaining collection times begins when the patient finishes drinking the glucose solution (see Table 5-1). Note this time. Outpatients are given a copy of the schedule and instructed to continue fasting, to drink water, and to remain in the drawing station area.

TABLE 5-1	Sample Oral Glucose Tolerance Test Schedule
Test Procedure	**3-Hour Test**
Fasting blood	0700
Patient finishes glucose	0800
1-hour sample	0900
2-hour sample	1000
3-hour sample	1100

Step 6. Collect remaining samples at the scheduled times. Timing of sample collection is critical, because test results are related to the scheduled times; any discrepancies should be noted on the requisition.

Step 7. The type of evacuated tubes used for blood collection must be consistent. Blood samples that will not be tested until the end of the sequence should be collected in gray stopper tubes. Consistency of venipuncture

(Reproduced with permission from Strasinger, S.K., and Di Lorenzo, M.S.: The Phlebotomy Textbook, ed. 3. Philadelphia, F.A. Davis, 2011.)

or dermal puncture must also be maintained because glucose values differ between the two types of blood. Venous blood samples are preferred.

Step 8. Corresponding labels containing routinely required information and sample order in the test sequence, such as 1-hour, 2-hour, and 3-hour, are placed on the blood samples.

Step 9. During scheduled sample collections, blood collectors should also observe patients for any changes in their condition, such as dizziness, which might indicate a reaction to the glucose, and should report any changes to a supervisor.

Step 10. Some patients may not be able to tolerate the glucose solution, and if vomiting occurs, the time of the vomiting must be reported to a supervisor and the health-care provider contacted for a decision concerning whether to continue the test. Vomiting early in the procedure is considered the most critical, and in most situations, the tolerance test is discontinued.

Step 11. Transport samples to the laboratory immediately. Samples not collected in gray stopper tubes must be centrifuged or tested within 2 hours of collection for reliable results.

OGTT Preparation

Before the test, patients should be instructed to eat a balanced diet that includes 150 g per day of carbohydrates for 3 days and to fast for 8 hours but not more than 16 hours. **Box 5-2** lists medications that can interfere with the test results. For OGTTs, the fasting patient should be instructed to abstain from food and drinks (including coffee and unsweetened tea), except water, for

8 hours but not more than 16 hours before and during the test. Smoking, chewing tobacco, alcohol, sugarless gum, and vigorous exercise should be avoided before and during the test because they stimulate digestion and may cause inaccurate test results. Note on the requisition form if the patient is chewing gum. OGTT procedures should be scheduled to begin between 0700 and 0900, because glucose levels exhibit a diurnal variation.

BOX 5-2	Medications That May Interfere With OGTT

Alcohol
Anticonvulsants
Aspirin
Birth control pills
Blood pressure medications
Corticosteroids
Diuretics
Estrogen-replacement pills
Salicylates in high doses

2-Hour Oral Glucose Tolerance Test

The 2-hr OGTT requires the collection of a fasting glucose sample and having the patient drink a 75-g glucose solution within 5 minutes and return for a second glucose test in 2 hours. A result equal to or greater than 200 mg/dL is considered diagnostic of diabetes mellitus.

One- and Two-Step Methods for Gestational Diabetes

The one-step method used to diagnose gestational diabetes mellitus (GDM) uses the same procedure as does the diagnostic 2-hr OGTT except that blood is drawn and tested at both 1 hour and 2 hours after drinking the 75-g glucose solution, at 24 to 28 weeks of gestation in women not previously diagnosed with overt diabetes. The diagnosis of GDM is made when any of the following plasma glucose values are met or exceeded:

- Fasting: 92 mg/dL (5.1 mmol/L)
- 1 hr: 180 mg/dL (10.0 mmol/L)
- 2 hr: 153 mg/dL (8.5 mmol/L)

The two-step method requires the patient to receive two tests. In the first step, the nonfasting patient receives a 50-g glucose challenge, with plasma glucose testing performed at 1 hr. A value of equal to or less than 140 mg/dL is considered normal. If the plasma glucose level is equal to or greater than 140 mg/dL, step 2 is performed.

The second test is administered on a different day and consists of a 100-g, 3-hour OGTT when the patient is fasting. The diagnosis of GDM is made if at least two of the following are met or exceeded:

- Fasting: 95 mg/dL (5.3 mmol/L)
- 1 hr: 180 mg/dL (10.0 mmol/L)

- 2 hr: 155 mg/dL (8.6 mmol/L)
- 3 hr: 140 mg/dL (7.8 mmol/L)

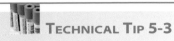

TECHNICAL TIP 5-3

Closely observe the patient for symptoms of hyperglycemia or hypoglycemia when collecting OGTT samples.

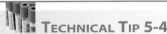

TECHNICAL TIP 5-4

Outpatients must understand the importance of adhering to the scheduled blood collection times for accurate results.

Diurnal Variation

In addition to glucose, other substances such as cortisol, testosterone, estradiol, progesterone, renin, thyroid-stimulating hormone (TSH), serum iron, and white blood cells (most often eosinophils) also exhibit **diurnal variation,** and the levels of these substances fluctuate noticeably throughout the day. Certain variations can be substantial. For example, plasma cortisol levels collected between 0800 and 1000 will be twice as high as levels collected at 1600, and serum iron levels collected in the morning are one-third higher than those collected in the evening. Samples must be collected at the specified time or the health-care provider should be notified and the test rescheduled for the next day.

Therapeutic Drug Monitoring

The blood levels of some therapeutic drugs are monitored to ensure safety and medication effectiveness. Frequently monitored drugs are listed in **Box 5-3.**

Random samples are occasionally requested; however, the most beneficial levels are the trough and peak levels. The **trough level** is collected 30 minutes before the next dose of medication is scheduled and represents the lowest level in the blood and ensures the drug is in the therapeutic range. Ideally, trough levels should be tested before administering the next dose to ensure that the level is low enough for the patient to receive more medication safely. The **peak level** is collected after medication administration at the time when the manufacturer

---

BOX 5-3 Frequently Monitored Therapeutic Drugs

Digoxin
Phenobarbital
Lithium
Gentamicin
Tobramycin
Vancomycin
Dilantin
Amikacin
Valproic acid
Theophylline
Methotrexate
Various antibiotics

---

specifies that the blood level should be at the highest point. The time of the peak level varies with the medication, the patient's metabolism, and the method of administration (30 minutes after IV, 1 hour after intramuscular, and 1 to 2 hours after oral doses) and ensures the drug is not at a toxic level. Information from drug manufacturers provides the half-life, the toxicity level, and the recommended times for collection of peak levels.

To ensure correct documentation of peak and trough levels, requisition forms and sample tube labels should include the time and method of administration of the last dose given, as well as the time that the sample is collected. Therapeutic drug monitoring collections must be coordinated with the pharmacy, laboratory, and nursing staff.

TECHNICAL TIP 5-5

Depending on the half-life of the medication, the timing of peak levels in therapeutic drug monitoring can be critical.

TECHNICAL TIP 5-6

Collection of blood in gel serum separator tubes has caused falsely low levels for certain medications. Red stopper tubes without the gel are recommended for therapeutic drug monitoring, and samples should be transported in an upright position.

BLOOD CULTURES

Blood cultures are requested to detect **septicemia** in febrile patients. Samples are usually collected in sets of two drawn either 30 or 60 minutes apart or just before the patient's temperature spikes. If antibiotics are to be started immediately, the sets are drawn at the same time from different sites. Samples collected from multiple sites at the same time serve as controls for possible contamination and must be labeled according to the collection site, such as right arm antecubital vein, and their number in the series (#1, #2). A known skin contaminant must be cultured from at least two of the sites for it to be considered a possible pathogen.

Blood for the culture may be drawn directly into bottles containing culture media using a winged blood collection set, transferred to the bottles from a syringe with a transfer device, or drawn into sterile, yellow stopper evacuated tubes containing anticoagulant and transferred to culture media in the laboratory. Each set should be collected in the same manner as the first set.

An anticoagulant must be present in the tube or the medium to prevent microorganisms from being trapped within a clot, where they might be undetected. The anticoagulant sodium polyanethol sulfonate (SPS) is used for blood cultures because it does not inhibit bacterial growth and may enhance it by inhibiting the action of phagocytes, complement, and some antibiotics. Other anticoagulants, such as sodium citrate, heparin, ethylenediaminetetraacetic acid (EDTA), or oxalate, should not be used because bacterial growth may be inhibited. Some blood culture collection systems have antimicrobial removal devices (ARDs) containing a resin that inactivates antibiotics. Blood culture bottles must be gently inverted eight times after the blood is added.

Blood cultures may be collected from IV lines by specially trained personnel (see Chapter 8). The recommended procedure is to collect one blood culture from the IV line and a second culture by venipuncture. Both sources must be documented according to the facility's policy.

⚠ SAFETY TIP 5-1

Occupational Safety & Health Administration (OSHA) regulations require using a blood transfer device for transferring the blood. The earlier practice of putting a new needle on the syringe to inoculate the blood culture bottle directly is no longer acceptable.

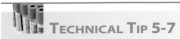

Collection With a Winged Blood Collection Set

A winged blood collection set with a Luer-Lock adapter and a specially designed holder can be used to transfer blood directly from the patient to bottles containing culture media. The Luer-Lock adapter on the winged blood collection apparatus attaches to the transfer device that contains a stopper-puncturing needle. Blood flows from the vein through the winged blood collection set tubing, Luer-Lock adapter, and stopper-puncturing needle into the culture bottle. Fill the aerobic bottle first because the winged blood collection set tubing has 0.5 mL of air in it. Keep the blood collection bottle lower than the collection site to prevent the culture media coming in contact with the stopper or needle during blood collection.

Collection With a Syringe

Blood can be collected in a syringe and aseptically transferred to blood culture bottles using a special transfer device. The anaerobic blood culture bottle must be filled first. The transfer device can then be adjusted to fit the size of other evacuated tubes for additional tests.

Cleansing the Site

Strict adherence to **aseptic** technique during sample collection is essential to ensure that a positive blood culture is not caused by external contamination. Antiseptics for disinfecting the blood collection site include 2 percent iodine tincture, 10 percent povidone-iodine, multiple 70 percent isopropyl alcohol preps, and chlorhexidine gluconate, and all are effective in killing bacteria on the skin when correctly used.

Two-Step Cleansing Procedure

The two-step procedure for cleansing the venipuncture site begins by scrubbing of the site with isopropyl alcohol for 30 to 60 seconds. The alcohol is followed by povidone-iodine or 2 percent iodine tincture applied by starting in the center of the site and progressing outward 3 to 4 inches in concentric circles. The povidone-iodine must be allowed to dry for 1 minute and the 2 percent iodine tincture for at least 30 seconds. To prevent irritation of the arm, remove the iodine with alcohol when the procedure is complete.

One-Step Cleansing Procedure

Chlorhexidine gluconate/isopropyl alcohol solution (ChloraPrep, Medi-Flex, Cardinal Health, Leawood, KS) is recommended because of its increased effectiveness in reducing blood culture contamination and the incidence of iodine sensitivity in patients. It is a one-step application using a commercially prepared swab or sponge. The venipuncture site is scrubbed for 30 to 60 seconds in a back-and-forth motion creating a friction on the skin, which is effective in skin antisepsis. Chlorhexidine gluconate is not recommended for infants younger than 2 months because of the risk of a chemical burn. Seventy percent isopropyl alcohol is recommended in this situation.

The site should not be repalpated after the venipuncture site has been cleaned; however, if the site must be touched after cleansing, the gloved palpating finger must be cleaned in the same manner as the site was prepared.

The tops of the collection containers also are cleaned before inoculating them with blood. The plastic caps are removed and the rubber stoppers are disinfected using 70 percent alcohol and covered with the alcohol pad until ready for inoculation.

Sample Collection

Two samples are routinely collected for each blood culture set, one to be incubated aerobically and the other to be incubated anaerobically. When a syringe is used, the anaerobic bottle should be inoculated first to prevent possible exposure to air. When the sample is collected using a winged blood collection set, the aerobic bottle is inoculated first so that the air in the tubing does not enter the anaerobic bottle. As with all syringe-to-tube transfers, a transfer device is used. Do not inoculate directly from the syringe to the bottle. Filling bottles directly through an evacuated tube needle and holder system is not recommended because of the possibility of culture media refluxing back into the vein. It also is difficult to ensure that the correct volume of blood has been collected. **Procedure 5-2** illustrates the steps in the blood culture procedure.

Procedure 5-2 Blood Culture Sample Collection Using a Syringe

Equipment:

Requisition form
Gloves
Tourniquet
Chlorhexidine gluconate (or other acceptable
    skin antiseptic)
Alcohol pads
Blood culture bottles
Syringe
Hypodermic needle with safety device or
    Point-Lok device

Blood transfer device
Winged blood collection set and tube holder
2 × 2 gauze
Sharps container
Indelible pen
Bandage
Biohazard bag

Procedure:

Step 1. Obtain and examine the requisition form.

Step 2. Greet the patient, explain the procedure to be performed, and obtain consent.

Step 3. Identify the patient following normal protocol.

Step 4. Prepare the patient and verify allergies.

Step 5. Select equipment.

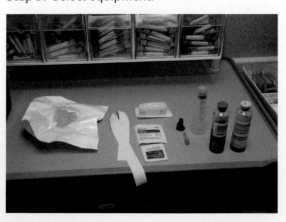

Step 6. Sanitize hands and put on gloves.

Step 7. Apply the tourniquet and locate the venipuncture site.

Step 8. Release tourniquet.

Step 9. Sterilize the site using chlorhexidine gluconate. Creating a friction, rub for 30 to 60 seconds and allow to air-dry for at least 30 seconds for antisepsis.

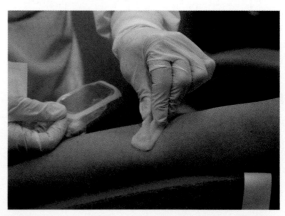

Step 10. Assemble equipment while the antiseptic is drying. Attach the needle to the syringe.

Procedure 5-2 Blood Culture Sample Collection Using a Syringe (Continued)

Step 11. Remove the plastic cap on the collection bottle. Confirm the volume of blood required from the label.

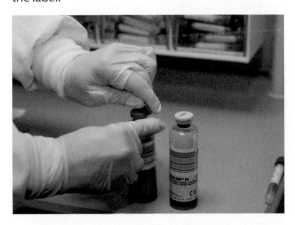

Step 12. Clean the top of the bottles with a 70 percent isopropyl alcohol pad and allow to dry.

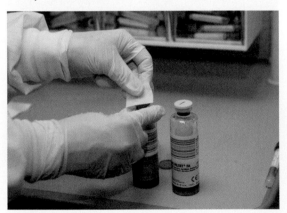

Step 13. Reapply the tourniquet and perform the venipuncture. Do not repalpate the site without cleansing the palpating finger in the same manner as the puncture site.

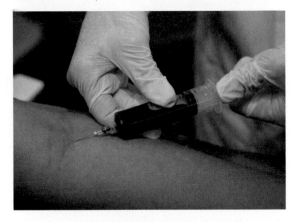

Step 14. Release the tourniquet. Place gauze over the puncture site, remove the needle, and apply pressure.

Step 15. Activate the safety device or remove the syringe needle with a Point-Lok device.

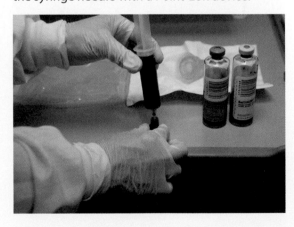

Step 16. Attach safety transfer device.

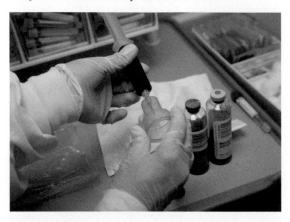

Step 17. Inoculate the anaerobic blood culture bottle first when using a syringe or second when using a winged blood collection set.

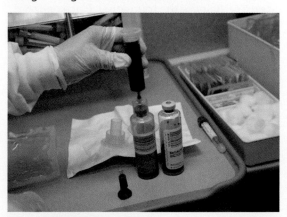

Step 18. Dispense the correct amount of blood into bottles. Some facilities require documenting the amount of blood dispensed.

Step 19. Mix the blood culture bottles by gentle inversion eight times.

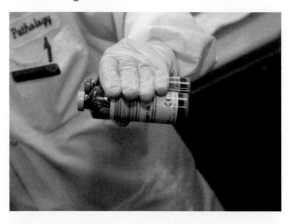

Step 20. Fill other collection tubes after the blood culture tubes.

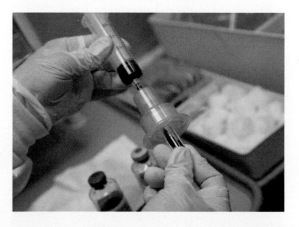

Step 21. Clean the iodine off the arm with alcohol if used.

| **PROCEDURE 5-2** **Blood Culture Sample Collection Using a Syringe** (Continued) |

Step 22. Label the samples appropriately and include the site of collection. Verify identification with the patient.

Step 23. Dispose of used equipment and supplies in a biohazard container.

Step 24. Check the venipuncture site for bleeding and bandage the patient's arm.

Step 25. Thank the patient, remove gloves, and sanitize hands.

(Reproduced with permission from Strasinger, S.K., and Di Lorenzo, M.S.: The Phlebotomy Textbook, ed. 3. Philadelphia, F.A. Davis, 2011.)

 TECHNICAL TIP 5-8

Follow the manufacturer's instructions when using commercially packaged venipuncture site blood culture prep kits.

A 1:10 ratio of blood to culture medium is critical because the number of microorganisms present in the blood is often small. Underfilled blood culture bottles may cause false-negative results. Overfilling of bottles should be avoided because this may cause false-positive results with automated systems. Adult blood culture bottles usually require 8 to 10 mL for each and pediatric bottles require 1 to 3 mL for each. Read the bottle label for the size of blood sample required. Pediatric blood culture volume requirements are based on the child's weight. Draw 1 mL of blood from babies weighing less than 5 kg, and place all the blood in one pediatric aerobic bottle.

ARTERIAL BLOOD GASES

Testing of arterial blood gases (ABGs) measures the ability of the lungs to provide oxygen (O_2) to the blood and to remove carbon dioxide (CO_2) from the blood and exhale it.

Conditions requiring the measurement of blood gases may be of respiratory or metabolic origin and include chronic obstructive pulmonary disease (COPD), cardiac and respiratory failures, severe shock, lung cancer, diabetic coma, open heart surgery, and respiratory distress syndrome (RDS) in premature infants. **Table 5-2** describes the tests and reference values for arterial blood gases.

A thorough understanding of arterial punctures and specialized training in the technique, precautions, complications, and sample handling is required. Instruction on performing arterial punctures must include supervised puncture performance under the supervision of a qualified instructor.

Patient Assessment

Patient information that must be recorded on the patient test requisition form includes the following:

- Time of collection
- Patient's temperature
- Patient's respiration rate
- Method of ventilation
- Amount of oxygen the patient is receiving
- Patient activity
- Collection site and method

The patient should have been receiving the specified amount of oxygen and have refrained from exercise for at least 20 to 30 minutes before obtaining the sample, defined as a **steady state.**

Arterial Puncture Sites

To be an acceptable puncture site, an artery must be:

- Large enough to accept at least a 25-gauge needle
- Located near the skin surface so that deep puncture is not required
- In an area where injury to surrounding tissues will not be critical
- Located in an area where other arteries are present to supply blood (collateral circulation) in case the punctured artery is damaged

TABLE 5-2 Arterial Blood Tests

Arterial Blood Test	Description/Function	Normal Values
Partial pressure of oxygen (Po$_2$)	Measures the pressure of O$_2$ dissolved in the blood. Tells how well O$_2$ moves from the lungs into the blood.	75–100 mm mercury (Hg)
Partial pressure of carbon dioxide (Pco$_2$)	Measures the pressure of CO$_2$ dissolved in the blood. Tells how well CO$_2$ moves out of the lungs.	35–45 mm Hg
pH	Measures the acidity or alkalinity of the blood. Indicates acidosis or alkalosis.	7.35–7.45
Bicarbonate (HCO$_3$)	Buffers the blood to prevent acidosis or alkalosis.	20–29 mEq/L
Oxygen content ($_{ct}$O$_2$)	Measures the amount of O$_2$ in the blood.	15–22 mL/100 mL of blood
Oxygen saturation (O$_2$ saturation)	Measures how much of the hemoglobin in the red blood cells is carrying O$_2$.	95%–100%

Reproduced with permission from Strasinger, S.K., and Di Lorenzo, M.S.: The Phlebotomy Textbook, ed. 3. Philadelphia, F.A. Davis, 2011.

Radial Artery

The radial artery, located on the thumb side of the wrist, is the artery of choice because the ulnar artery can provide collateral circulation to the hand if the radial artery is damaged. It lies close to the surface of the wrist and is easily accessible **(Fig. 5-1A).** The radial artery is easily compressed against the wrist ligaments, so that pressure can be applied more effectively on the puncture site after removal of the needle and there is less chance of a hematoma.

Brachial Artery

The brachial artery, located near the basilic vein, is sometimes used **(see Fig. 5-1A).** Because of its depth, its location near the basilic vein and median nerve, and the fact that it lies in soft tissue that does not provide adequate support for postpuncture pressure, it is not routinely used.

Femoral Artery

The femoral artery, located in the groin area of the leg, is the largest artery used for arterial puncture **(see Fig. 5-1B).** Only specially trained personnel may collect samples from the femoral artery because of its lack of collateral circulation. These are also the only personnel authorized to insert and collect samples from arterial cannulas.

Modified Allen Test

Before performing a radial artery puncture, the Modified Allen Test is performed to determine whether the ulnar artery is capable of providing collateral circulation to the hand. Lack of available circulation could result in loss of the hand or its function, and another site should be chosen. The Modified Allen Test is shown in **Procedure 5-3**.

Preparing the Site

The puncture site is cleansed with alcohol and the area is allowed to air-dry. A local anesthetic may be administered at this time. This is done by injecting a small amount of 1 percent lidocaine without epinephrine just under the skin, or into the surrounding tissue if the artery is deep. Before injecting the anesthetic, gently pull back on the plunger and check for the appearance of blood, which would indicate that a blood vessel rather than tissue has been entered. If blood appears in the syringe, a new syringe must be prepared and a slightly different injection site must be chosen. Allow 2 minutes for the anesthetic to take effect, and if the patient is apprehensive, allow him or her to relax for 5 minutes.

Performing the Puncture

Using a preassembled syringe with a safety needle, set the syringe plunger to the correct fill level. Just before performing the puncture, the artery is relocated with the cleansed finger of the nondominant hand. The

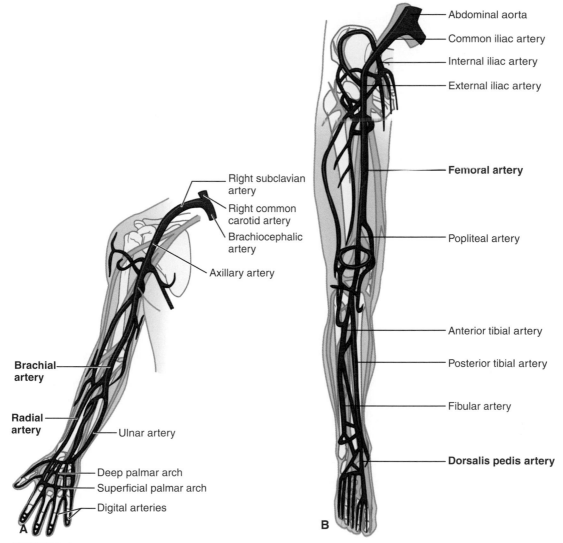

FIGURE 5-1 *A, Arteries in the arm. B, Arteries in the leg.* *(Reproduced with permission from Strasinger, SK, and Di Lorenzo, MS: The Phlebotomy Textbook, ed. 3. Philadelphia, FA Davis, 2011.)*

finger is placed directly over the area where the needle should enter the artery, not where the needle enters the skin.

The heparinized syringe is held like dart in the dominant hand and the needle is inserted about 5 to 10 mm below the palpating finger at a 30- to 45-degree angle with the bevel up. The needle is slowly advanced into the artery until blood appears in the needle hub. At this time, arterial pressure should cause blood to pump into the syringe. The plunger may have to be very carefully pulled back when a smaller than 23-gauge needle is used. If blood does not appear, the needle may be slightly redirected but must remain under the skin.

 TECHNICAL TIP 5-9

Blood that does not pulse into the syringe and appears dark rather than bright red may be venous blood and should not be used.

Needle Removal

When enough blood has been collected, remove the needle and apply firm pressure to the site with a gauze pad for a minimum of 3 to 5 minutes. Application of

PROCEDURE 5-3 The Modified Allen Test

EQUIPMENT:

None

PROCEDURE:

Step 1. Extend the patient's wrist over a rolled towel and ask the patient to form a tight fist.

Step 2. Locate the pulses of the radial and ulnar arteries on the palmar surface of the wrist by palpating with the second and third fingers, not the thumb, which has a pulse.

Step 3. Compress both arteries.

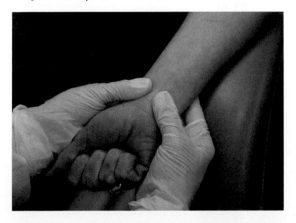

Step 4. Have the patient open the fist and observe that the palm has become pale (blanched).

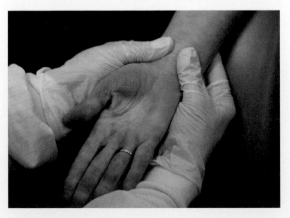

Step 5. Release pressure on the ulnar artery only and watch to see that color returns to the palm. This should occur within 15 seconds if the ulnar artery is functioning (Positive Modified Allen Test).

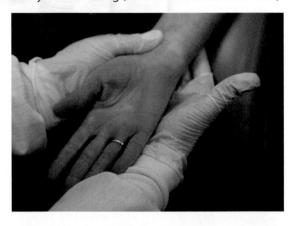

Step 6. If color does not appear (negative Modified Allen Test), the radial artery must not be used. If the Modified Allen Test is positive, proceed by palpating the radial artery to determine its depth, direction, and size.

(Modified with permission from Strasinger, S.K., and Di Lorenzo, M.S.: The Phlebotomy Textbook, ed. 3. Philadelphia, F.A. Davis, 2011.)

PROCEDURE 5-4 Preparing and Administering the Local Anesthetic

EQUIPMENT:

Gloves
25- or 26- gauge needle
1-mL syringe

1 percent lidocaine without epinephrine
Alcohol wipes
Sharps container

PROCEDURE:

1. Greet the patient, explain the procedure to be performed, and obtain consent.
2. Sanitize hands and put on gloves.
3. Attach needle to syringe.
4. Cleanse the vial top of the lidocaine bottle with alcohol.
5. Insert the needle into the top of the bottle and withdraw 0.5 mL of lidocaine.
6. Recap the needle and place it horizontally on the table.
7. Locate and cleanse the puncture site with alcohol and allow the site to air-dry.
8. Using the nondominant hand, raise the skin slightly above the artery puncture site.
9. Insert the needle into the raised skin at approximately a 10-degree angle.
10. Slightly pull back on the syringe plunger before injecting the lidocaine to be sure that blood does not appear because that would indicate puncture of a blood vessel.
11. Slowly inject the lidocaine, forming a raised wheal.
12. Remove the needle and allow 2 to 3 minutes for the anesthesia to take effect.
13. Record the administration of the lidocaine on the requisition form.
14. Proceed with the arterial puncture procedure when the patient has relaxed.

---

pressure for longer than 5 minutes may be necessary for patients receiving anticoagulant therapy. If bleeding has not stopped, reapply pressure for an additional 2 minutes and check for hemostasis. Continue this process until the bleeding has stopped.

Removing the Air and Mixing Sample

With the hand holding the syringe, immediately expel any air that has entered the sample. Activate the needle safety shield, remove the needle, and apply the Luer-Lok cap or insert the needle into an approved safety device. Immediately rotate or invert the syringe to mix the anticoagulant with the entire sample.

Completion of the Procedure

When both hands are free, the sample is labeled. After pressure has been removed for 2 minutes, the patient's arm is rechecked to be sure that a hematoma is not forming, in which case additional pressure is required.

The radial artery is checked for a pulse below the puncture site, and the nurse or health-care provider is notified if a pulse cannot be located. This would indicate a possible **arteriospasm.**

A pressure bandage is applied if no complications are discovered. Before leaving the room, dispose of used materials in appropriate containers, remove gloves, sanitize hands, and thank the patient. **Procedure 5-5** describes the steps involved in performing the arterial puncture.

Sample Integrity

ABG test results can be noticeably affected by improper sample collection and handling. **Table 5-3** describes technical errors that will affect sample integrity.

CLSI recommendations state that samples that will be analyzed within 30 minutes should be collected in plastic syringes and not placed in an ice slurry unless a lactic acid test has been ordered with the ABG, which must be placed in an ice slurry immediately.

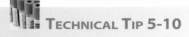

TECHNICAL TIP 5-10

Samples that will also have electrolytes performed cannot be placed in an ice slurry.

PROCEDURE 5-5 Radial Artery Puncture

EQUIPMENT:

Requisition form
Gloves
Antiseptic (iodine or chlorhexidine)
Alcohol pads
Heparinized syringe
Needle with safety device
Luer-Lock cap

Gauze pads
Self-adhesive pressure bandage
Ice slurry, if necessary
Indelible pen
Sharps container
Biohazard bag

PROCEDURE:

Step 1. Obtain a requisition form and check for completeness.

Step 2. Greet and identify the patient.

Step 3. Explain the procedure, reassure the patient, and obtain informed consent.

Step 4. Obtain oxygen therapy information and ensure a steady state.

Step 5. Sanitize hands and put on gloves.

Step 6. Organize equipment.

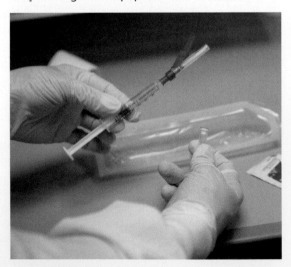

Step 7. Heparinize a glass syringe and prepare the local anesthesia syringe if necessary.

Step 8. Support and hyperextend the patient's wrist.

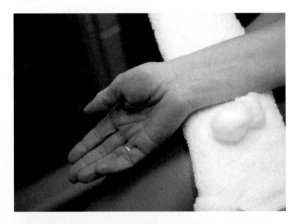

Step 9. Perform the Modified Allen Test.

Step 10. Locate and palpate the radial artery.

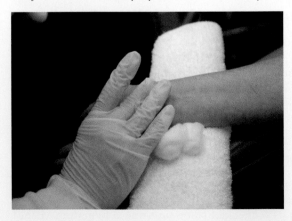

PROCEDURE 5-5 **Radial Artery Puncture** (Continued)

Step 11. Cleanse the site and the palpating finger.

Step 12. Administer anesthetic if necessary.

Step 13. Place a clean, gloved finger over the arterial puncture site.

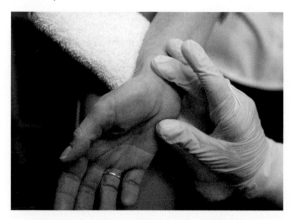

Step 14. Insert needle, bevel up at a 30- to 45-degree angle, 10 to 15 mm below the palpating finger.

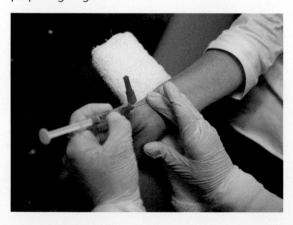

Step 15. Allow syringe to fill.

Step 16. Remove needle and apply pressure.

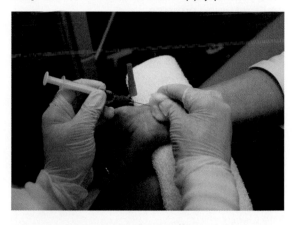

Step 17. Activate safety shield, maintaining pressure.

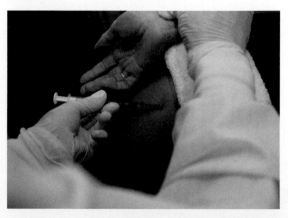

Step 18. Remove needle while retaining pressure.

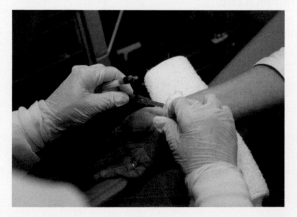

PROCEDURE 5-5 Radial Artery Puncture (Continued)

Step 19. Apply Luer device and mix syringe while retaining pressure.

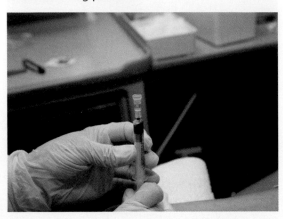

Step 20. Check puncture site for bleeding after 3 to 5 minutes. Maintain pressure if bleeding has not stopped.

(Modified with permission from Strasinger, S.K., and Di Lorenzo, M.S.: The Phlebotomy Textbook, ed. 3. Philadelphia, F.A. Davis, 2011.)

Step 21. Label sample after bleeding has stopped.

Step 22. Reexamine puncture site.

Step 23. Check for radial pulse.

Step 24. Apply pressure bandage.

Step 25. Remove gloves and sanitize hands.

Step 26. Thank patient.

Step 27. Immediately deliver sample to the laboratory.

TABLE 5-3 Effect of Technical Errors on Arterial Blood Gas Results

Technical Error	Effect
Air bubbles present	Atmospheric oxygen enters the sample, and carbon dioxide from the sample enters the air bubbles.
Too much heparin	pH is lowered.
Too little heparin/inadequate mixing	The presence of clots will interfere with the analyzer.
Delayed analysis	White blood cells and platelets in the sample continue their metabolism, utilizing oxygen and producing carbon dioxide.
Venous rather than arterial sample	There is a falsely decreased P_{O_2} and increased P_{CO_2}.

Reproduced with permission from Strasinger, S.K., and Di Lorenzo, M.S.: The Phlebotomy Textbook, ed. 3. Philadelphia, F.A. Davis, 2011.

Arterial Puncture Complications

The arterial puncture is more dangerous for the patient than the venipuncture. **Table 5-4** describes possible complications and how they can be prevented.

SPECIAL SAMPLE HANDLING PROCEDURES

Instructions for the collection, transportation, and storage of all laboratory samples are available from the laboratory and should be strictly followed to maintain sample integrity. Some tests require that the sample be kept warm, chilled, frozen, or protected from light.

Cold Agglutinins

Cold agglutinins are autoantibodies produced by persons infected with *Mycoplasma pneumoniae* or autoimmune hemolytic anemia. The autoantibodies react with red blood cells (RBCs) at temperatures below body temperature.

Because the cold agglutinins in the serum attach to RBCs when the blood cools to below body temperature, the sample must be kept warm until the serum can be separated from the cells. Samples are collected in tubes that have been warmed in an incubator at 37°C for 30 minutes and that contain no additives or gels that could interfere with the test. The warmed tube is carried to the patient's room in the blood collector's tightly closed fist or a prewarmed container. The sample is collected as quickly as possible and immediately delivered to the laboratory in the same manner and placed in the incubator. Failure to keep a sample warm prior to

serum separation produces falsely decreased test results. Cryofibrinogen and cryoglobulin are two proteins that precipitate when cold and must be collected and handled in the same manner as cold agglutinins.

TECHNICAL TIP 5-11

The CLSI recommends not to ice arterial blood gases (ABGs) when they have been collected in plastic syringes and analyzed within 30 minutes unless they are collected in conjunction with lactic acid.

Chilled Samples

Chilling a sample inhibits metabolic processes that continue after blood collection and can adversely affect laboratory results. Examples of samples that require chilling to prevent deterioration are shown in **Box 5-4**.

For adequate chilling, the sample must be placed in a mixture of crushed ice and water at the bedside or in a uniform ice block **(see Fig. 5-2)**. Placing a sample in or on ice cubes is not acceptable, because uniform chilling will not occur. It is important that these samples be immediately delivered to the laboratory for processing.

TECHNICAL TIP 5-12

Bilirubin is rapidly destroyed in samples exposed to light and can decrease up to 50 percent after 1 hour of exposure to light.

TABLE 5-4 Arterial Puncture Complications

Complication	Cause	Prevention
Hematoma	Arterial blood entering the tissue	Blood collector applies pressure until bleeding stops
Tissue destruction/gangrene	Arteriospasm	Evaluate collateral circulation
Vasovagal reaction	Apprehension/pain	Calming the patient, local anesthetic
Hemorrhage	Coagulation disorders and thrombolytic therapy	Increased pressure, smaller-gauge needles
Infection	Failure to adequately cleanse the site	Proper cleansing, sterile technique
Nerve damage	Deep punctures	Avoiding deep sites or additional training for deep sites

Reproduced with permission from Strasinger, S.K., and Di Lorenzo, M.S.: The Phlebotomy Textbook, ed. 3. Philadelphia, F.A. Davis, 2011.

> ## BOX 5-4　Examples of Analytes That May Require Chilling
>
> Ammonia
> Lactic acid
> Acetone
> Free fatty acids
> Pyruvate
> Glucagon
> Gastrin
> Adrenocorticotropic hormone (ACTH)
> Parathyroid hormone (PTH)
> Renin
> Angiotensin-converting enzyme (ACE)
> Catecholamines
> Homocysteine
> Some coagulation studies
> Arterial blood gases (only if indicated)

> ## BOX 5-5　Analytes Sensitive to Light
>
> Bilirubin
> Beta-carotene
> Vitamin A
> Vitamin B_6
> Vitamin B_{12}
> Folate
> Porphyrins

Samples Sensitive to Light

Exposure to artificial light or sunlight (ultraviolet) for any length of time may decrease the concentration of various analytes that are listed in **Box 5-5**. Wrapping the tubes in aluminum foil or using an amber-colored transport tube can protect samples **(see Fig. 5-3)**. Tubes

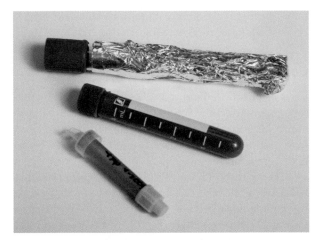

FIGURE 5-3　Analytes protected from light. *(Reprinted with permission from Strasinger, S.K., and Di Lorenzo, M.S.: The Phlebotomy Textbook, ed. 3. Philadelphia, F.A. Davis, 2011.)*

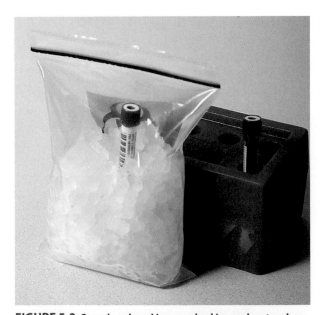

FIGURE 5-2　Samples placed in a crushed ice and water slurry and an ice block. *(Reprinted with permission from Strasinger, S.K., and Di Lorenzo, M.S.: The Phlebotomy Textbook, ed. 3. Philadelphia, F.A. Davis, 2011.)*

should be kept closed. Refer to Chapter 1 for proper preparation and transport of samples from off-site collection facilities.

Sample Storage

To prevent contamination of plasma and serum by cellular constituents, it is recommended that samples be separated within 2 hours. Anticoagulated samples can be centrifuged immediately after collection, and the plasma removed. Samples collected without anticoagulant must be fully clotted before centrifugation. Samples for hematology whole blood analysis should never be centrifuged.

Based on the tests requested, separated serum or plasma may remain at room temperature for 8 hours. If testing has not been completed in 8 hours, the specimen should be refrigerated. If testing is not complete in 48 hours, the serum or plasma should be frozen. Refer to the laboratory procedure manual for specific analyte instructions.

The Clinical and Laboratory Standards Institute (CLSI) GP44-A4 guideline recommends time limits for testing of samples. Examples include the following:

- Coagulation samples for activated partial thromboplastin times (APTTs) are stable at room temperature for 4 hours unless the patient is on heparin, in which case the plasma must be removed from the cells within 1 hour after collection and tested within 4 hours.
- Samples for prothrombin time (PT) testing are stable for 24 hours at room temperature.
- All other coagulation tests must be performed within 4 hours of collection. When samples cannot be assayed within the required time frame, the platelet-poor plasma must be separated from the red cells and frozen within 1 hour of collection.
- Blood smears from EDTA tubes must be made within 1 hour of collection to avoid cell distortion and artifact caused by the EDTA anticoagulant.
- EDTA samples for complete blood counts (CBCs) are stable for 24 hours at room temperature; however, for certain manufacturer's tubes, CBCs should be analyzed within 6 hours. EDTA samples for CBCs collected in microcollection containers must be tested in 4 hours.
- ESR tests must be performed within 4 hours in EDTA samples stored at room temperature and or within 12 hours when refrigerated.
- Reticulocyte counts collected in EDTA should be analyzed within 6 hours when stored at room temperature or up to 72 hours when refrigerated.
- Samples for glucose tests collected in sodium fluoride tubes are stable for 24 hours at room temperature and 48 hours when refrigerated.

Legal Samples

The **chain of custody** must be followed exactly when drawing samples for test results that may be used as evidence in legal proceedings. Special forms are provided for the documentation of sample handling, and special containers and seals may be required **(see Fig. 5-4).** Documentation must include the date, time, and identification of each person handling the sample. Samples should not be left sitting on a counter unattended. Patient identification and sample collection should take place in the presence of a witness, often a law enforcement officer. Identification requires specific documents and may require photographs, fingerprints, or heel prints. The tests requested most frequently are alcohol and drug levels and DNA analysis.

TECHNICAL TIP 5-13

Technical errors and failure to follow chain-of-custody protocol are primary targets of the defense in legal proceedings.

Blood Alcohol Samples

When collecting samples for blood alcohol levels, the site should be cleansed with soap and water or a nonalcoholic antiseptic solution, such as benzalkonium chloride. To prevent the escape of the volatile alcohol into the atmosphere, tubes should be filled completely and not uncapped prior to delivery to the laboratory. Blood alcohol levels are frequently collected in gray stopper tubes; however, laboratory protocol should be strictly followed.

TECHNICAL TIP 5-14

Skin disinfectants such as tincture of iodine and chlorhexidine gluconate contain alcohol and should not be used to clean the site for a blood alcohol level.

Saint Joseph Hospital Toxicology Laboratory
601 N. 30th Street
Omaha, NE 68131-2197
(402) 449-4940

Drug Testing Custody & Control Form
NON-DOT/NON-HHS (NON-NIDA)

SPECIMEN ID NO. _____   LABORATORY ACCESSION NO. _____

▶ **STEP 1: TO BE COMPLETED BY COLLECTOR OR EMPLOYER REPRESENTATIVE**

A. Name, Address and I.D. No.   B. MRO Name and Address

C. Tests to be Performed: ☐ DS1   ☐ DS2   ☐ NON-NIDA5   ☐ URINE ALCOHOL   ☐ BLOOD ALCOHOL

D. Reason for Test: ☐ pre-employment ☐ current employment ☐ periodic ☐ reasonable susp/cause ☐ post accident ☐ other _____
                                                                                                                    specify

E. Donor I.D. _____

▶ **STEP 2: TO BE COMPLETED BY COLLECTOR -** Specimen temperature must be read within 4 minutes of collection.

Specimen temperature within range: ☐ Yes, 90.5° - 99.8°F/32.5° - 37.7°C   ☐ No, Record specimen temperature here _____

▶ **STEP 3: TO BE COMPLETED BY COLLECTOR AND DONOR -** Collector affixes bottle seal(s) to bottle(s). Collector dates seal(s). Donor initials seal(s).

▶ **STEP 4: TO BE COMPLETED BY DONOR -** Go to copy 2 (pink page); STEP 4.

▶ **STEP 5: TO BE COMPLETED BY COLLECTOR**

COLLECTION SITE LOCATION:

_____   (_____) _____
              Collection Facility   Collector's Business Phone No.

_____   _____ _____ _____
              Address   City   State   Zip

REMARKS:
_I certify that the specimen identified on this form is the specimen presented to me by the donor providing the certification on Copy 2 of this form, that it bears the same specimen identification
number as that set forth above, and that it has been collected, labeled and sealed._   AM
                                                   X   /   /   PM
_____   _____   _____   _____
(PRINT) Collector's Name (First, MI, Last)   Signature of Collector   Date (Mo./Day/Yr.)   Time

▶ **STEP 6: TO BE INITIATED BY THE COLLECTOR AND COMPLETED AS NECESSARY THEREAFTER**

DATE MO. DAY YR.	SPECIMEN RELEASED BY	SPECIMEN RECEIVED BY	PURPOSE OF CHANGE
/ /	**DONOR - NO SIGNATURE**	Signature _____ Name _____	PROVIDE SPECIMEN FOR TESTING
/ /	Signature _____ Name _____	Signature ~~Courier~~ Name _____	TRANSPORT TO LABORATORY
/ /	Signature ~~Courier~~ Name _____	Signature _____ Name _____	

– **INTENTIONALLY LEFT BLANK** –

_____
Date (Mo. Day. Yr.)

_____
Donor's Initials

PLACE OVER CAP

SPECIMEN ID NO. _____

_____
Date (Mo. Day. Yr.)

_____
Donor's Initials

PLACE OVER CAP

SPECIMEN ID NO. _____

TRANSPORT BOX CUSTODY SEAL

COLLECTOR'S INITIALS _____ DATE _____

COPY 1 - ORIGINAL - MUST ACCOMPANY SPECIMEN TO LABORATORY

FIGURE 5-4 Sample chain-of-custody form. *(Courtesy of Creighton University Medical Center, Omaha, NE. Reprinted with permission from Strasinger, S.K., and Di Lorenzo, M.S.: The Phlebotomy Textbook, ed. 3. Philadelphia, F.A. Davis, 2011.)*

BIBLIOGRAPHY

American Diabetes Association: Classification and Diagnosis of Diabetes. *Diabetes Care* 38(Suppl. 1):S8–S16, 2015.

CLSI: *Procedures for the Collection of Diagnostic Blood Specimens by Venipuncture*, ed. 6. Approved Guideline GP41-A6 (H03-A6). Wayne, PA, CLSI, 2007.

CLSI: *Collection, Transport, and Processing of Blood Specimens for Testing Plasma-Based Coagulation Assays and Molecular Hemostasis Assays*, ed. 2 Approved Standard H21-A5. Wayne, PA, CLSI, 2012.

CLSI: *Procedures for the Handling and Processing of Blood Specimens for Common Laboratory Tests*, ed. 4. Approved Guideline GP44-A4 (H18-A4). Wayne, PA, CLSI, 2012.

Emergency Nurses Association: *Clinical Practice Guideline: Prevention of Blood Culture Contamination*. December 2012.

National Committee for Clinical Laboratory Standards. *Procedures for the Collections of Arterial Blood Specimens*. Approved Guideline GP43-A4 (H11-A4). Wayne, PA, NCCLS/CLSI, 2004.

Strasinger, S.K., and DiLorenzo, M.S.: *The Phlebotomy Textbook*, ed. 3. Philadelphia, F.A. Davis, 2011.

INTERNET RESOURCES

www.clsi.org

www.cap.org

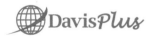 For additional material, please visit **http://davisplus.fadavis .com.**

REVIEW QUESTIONS

1. **The timing for a glucose tolerance test begins when:**
   a. The fasting sample is drawn
   b. The test results are completed on the fasting sample
   c. The patient finishes drinking the glucose
   d. 30 minutes has passed after the patient finished drinking the glucose

2. **When are samples scheduled for collection at specific times?**
   a. Measuring the body's metabolism of the test substance
   b. The substance exhibits diurnal variation
   c. To determine blood levels of medications prior to the next dose
   d. All of the above

3. **The trough level for therapeutic drug monitoring is collected:**
   a. 30 minutes after the medication is administered
   b. 30 minutes before the medication is administered
   c. At the time specified by the manufacturer
   d. After the patient has fasted for 8 hours

4. **A negative Modified Allen Test indicates:**
   a. The ulnar artery can be punctured
   b. The radial artery can be punctured
   c. The radial artery cannot be punctured
   d. No collateral circulation by the radial artery

5. **The preferred site for arterial puncture is the:**
   a. Brachial artery
   b. Ulnar artery
   c. Femoral artery
   d. Radial artery

6. **Two blood culture sets from a patient requiring STAT administration of antibiotics are collected:**
   a. 30 minutes apart
   b. Before and after the antibiotic is administered
   c. Immediately from two different sites
   d. Before and after the fever spikes

7. **When blood is inoculated into blood culture bottles using a winged blood collection set the:**
   a. Anaerobic bottle is inoculated first
   b. Safety device is activated first
   c. Aerobic bottle is inoculated first
   d. Volume of blood inoculated is increased

8. **Samples that require chilling immediately after collection are placed in a:**
   a. Container of ice cubes
   b. Container of crushed ice and water
   c. Bag of dry ice
   d. Flask of cold water

9. **Samples for cold agglutinins must be:**
   a. Transported on ice
   b. Drawn into a green stopper tube
   c. Processed in a refrigerated centrifuge
   d. Kept warm

10. **A falsely decreased blood alcohol level may be obtained if:**
    a. Blood is collected in a gray stopper tube
    b. The site is cleansed with Zephiran Chloride
    c. The tube is only partially filled
    d. The tube is overfilled

FOR FURTHER STUDY

1. Explain why collecting every other sample for a 3-hour OGTT by dermal puncture on an elderly patient would be unacceptable.

2. Would leaving a green stopper tube for a bilirubin test on the counter for 1 hour affect the result? Why? What is the correct procedure?

3. Why should the fasting glucose sample be tested before administering the glucose in an OGTT?

4. What instructions should be given to a patient prior to having blood drawn for a lipid panel?

CASE STUDY 1

Two sets of blood cultures that each consist of an aerobic and an anaerobic bottle are drawn from Mr. Jones 1 hour apart. The first set is drawn using a syringe and the second set using a winged blood collection set.

1. Is this a common pattern for blood cultures? Why or why not?

2. What error in technique could cause a positive anaerobic culture from the first set and a negative anaerobic culture in the second set?

3. What is the significance of a known skin contaminant growing in the aerobic bottle from the first set and not in the aerobic bottle from the second set?

4. Would failure to mix the bottles after the blood is added most probably cause a false-positive or false-negative culture?

CASE STUDY 2

Mary was having a difficult time collecting blood from the antecubital area of an obese patient. After redirecting the needle three or four times, Mary noticed that blood was pulsating into evacuated tube.

1. What other observation should Mary make?

2. What blood vessel may have been punctured?

3. What additional precautions should Mary take to protect the patient?

4. What is the most probable complication for this patient?

EVALUATION OF BLOOD CULTURE COLLECTION TECHNIQUE

RATING SYSTEM

2 = Satisfactory

1 = Needs improvement

0 = Incorrect/did not perform

_____ 1. Obtains and examines requisition.

_____ 2. Greets patient, explains the procedure to be performed, and obtains informed consent.

_____ 3. Identifies the patient verbally by stating the first and last name, DOB, and compares the information on the patient's ID band with the requisition form.

_____ 4. Sanitizes hands and applies gloves.

_____ 5. Applies tourniquet.

_____ 6. Selects puncture site.

_____ 7. Releases tourniquet.

_____ 8. Scrubs site with chlorhexidine gluconate for 30 to 60 seconds in a back-and-forth motion creating a friction.

_____ 9. Allows chlorhexidine gluconate to dry.

_____ 10. Assembles equipment.

_____ 11. Cleanses top of blood culture bottles with alcohol.

_____ 12. Reapplies tourniquet.

_____ 12. Does not retouch puncture site.

_____ 13. Performs venipuncture using a winged blood collection set or syringe.

_____ 14. Releases tourniquet.

_____ 15. Removes needle and activates safety device and applies pressure to site.

_____ 16. Disposes of needle in sharps container.

_____ 17. Inoculates anaerobic container first from syringe using a transfer device or second from winged blood collection set.

_____ 18. Dispenses correct amount of blood into bottles.

_____ 19. Mixes bottles by gentle inversion eight times.

_____ 20. Labels the samples and verifies information with the patient.

_____ 21. Disposes of used equipment and supplies in appropriate containers.

_____ 22. Checks puncture site for bleeding and bandages the patient's arm.

_____ 23. Thanks the patient, removes gloves, and sanitizes hands.

TOTAL POINTS

MAXIMUM POINTS = 46

COMMENTS:

EVALUATION OF MODIFIED ALLEN TEST

RATING SYSTEM

2 = Satisfactory

1 = Needs improvement

3 = 0 Incorrect/did not perform

_____ 1. Obtains and examines requisition.

_____ 2. Greets and identifies the patient verbally by stating the first and last name, DOB, and compares the information on the patient's ID band with the requisition form.

_____ 3. Explains procedure, reassures the patient, and obtains informed consent.

_____ 4. Extends patient's wrist and asks the patient to form a tight fist.

_____ 5. Locates the pulses of radial and ulnar arteries using appropriate fingers.

_____ 6. Compresses both arteries.

_____ 7. Asks patient to open the fist.

_____ 8. Looks for blanching of patient's palm.

_____ 9. Tells patient to leave hand open.

_____ 10. Releases pressure on the ulnar artery only.

_____ 11. Observes color of patient's palm within 15 seconds.

_____ 12. States whether the test is positive or negative.

_____ 13. Explains the significance of the test results.

TOTAL POINTS

MAXIMUM POINTS = 26

COMMENTS:

EVALUATION OF RADIAL ARTERY PUNCTURE

RATING SYSTEM

2 = Satisfactory

1 = Needs improvement

0 = Incorrect/did not perform

_____ 1. Obtains and examines requisition form.

_____ 2. Greets and identifies the patient verbally by stating the first and last name, DOB, and compares the information on the patient's ID band with the requisition form.

_____ 3. Explains the procedure, reassures the patient, and obtains informed consent.

_____ 4. Determines that the patient is in a steady state.

_____ 5. Obtains metabolic and oxygen therapy information.

_____ 6. Sanitizes hands and puts on gloves.

_____ 7. Organizes equipment.

_____ 8. Prepares anesthetic syringe if using.

_____ 9. Supports and hyperextends the patient's wrist.

_____ 10. Performs and interprets the Modified Allen Test.

_____ 11. Locates and palpates the radial artery.

_____ 12. Cleanses the site and allows it to air-dry.

_____ 13. Cleanses palpating finger.

_____ 14. Administers local anesthetic and waits 2 minutes if using.

_____ 15. Places a clean, gloved finger over puncture site.

_____ 16. Inserts needle, bevel up, at a 30- to 45-degree angle, 10 to 15 mm below palpating finger.

_____ 17. Allows syringe to fill by arterial pressure.

_____ 18. Removes needle and applies pressure.

_____ 19. Expels air bubbles from sample.

_____ 20. Activates needle safety device.

_____ 21. Removes needle from syringe and applies Luer-Lock device.

_____ 22. Rotates or inverts syringe to mix while maintaining pressure.

_____ 23. Examines puncture site after 3 to 5 minutes.

_____ 24. Disposes of needle in sharps container.

_____ 25. Labels sample.

_____ 26. Reexamines patient's arm.

_____ 27. Checks for a radial pulse.

_____ 28. Applies pressure bandage.

_____ 29. Disposes of used supplies in the appropriate containers.

_____ 30. Removes gloves and sanitizes hands.

_____ 31. Thanks patient.

_____ 32. Immediately delivers sample to the laboratory.

TOTAL POINTS

MAXIMUM POINTS = 64

COMMENTS:

6

Dermal Puncture

INTRODUCTION

Advances in laboratory instrumentation and the popularity of point-of-care testing have made it possible to perform a majority of laboratory tests on **microsamples** of blood obtained by dermal puncture on both pediatric and adult patients. This chapter presents the required equipment and correct procedure necessary for dermal punctures to provide quality samples.

Dermal puncture is the method of choice for collecting blood from infants and children younger than 2 years of age. Locating superficial veins large enough to accept even a small-gauge needle is difficult in these patients, and veins that are available may need to be reserved for IV therapy. Use of deep veins, such as the femoral vein, can be dangerous and may cause complications including cardiac arrest, venous thrombosis, hemorrhage, damage to surrounding tissue and organs, infection, reflex arteriospasm (which can possibly result in gangrene), and injury caused by restraining the child. Drawing excessive amounts of blood from premature and small infants can rapidly cause anemia, because a 2-lb infant may have a total blood volume of only 150 mL.

In adults, dermal puncture may be required for a variety of reasons, including the following:

1. Burned or scarred patients
2. Patients receiving chemotherapy who require frequent tests and whose veins must be reserved for therapy
3. Patients with thrombotic tendencies
4. Geriatric or other patients with very fragile veins
5. Patients with inaccessible veins
6. Home glucose monitoring and point-of-care testing

It may not be possible to obtain a satisfactory sample by **dermal** puncture from patients who are severely dehydrated, have poor peripheral circulation, or have swollen fingers. The **interstitial fluid** in a swollen finger may dilute the blood sample if a finger puncture is performed. Certain tests may not be collected by dermal puncture because of the larger amount of blood required; these include some coagulation studies, erythrocyte sedimentation rates, and blood cultures.

IMPORTANCE OF CORRECT COLLECTION

Correct collection techniques are critical because of the smaller amount of blood that is collected and the higher possibility of sample contamination, microclots, and hemolysis. Hemolysis is more frequently seen in samples collected by dermal puncture than it is in those collected by venipuncture and may be caused by:

- Excessive squeezing ("milking") of the puncture site to obtain enough blood
- Increased numbers and fragility of red blood cells (RBCs) in newborns
- Residual alcohol at the site
- Vigorous mixing of the microcollection tubes after collection

The presence of hemolysis may not be detected in samples containing bilirubin, but it interferes not only with the tests routinely affected by hemolysis, but also with the frequently requested neonatal bilirubin determination.

Composition of Capillary Blood

Blood collected by dermal puncture comes from the capillaries, arterioles, and venules and may also contain small amounts of tissue (interstitial) fluid. Because of arterial pressure, the composition of this blood more closely resembles arterial blood than venous blood. With the exception of arterial blood gases (ABGs), few chemical differences exist between arterial and venous blood. The concentration of glucose is higher in blood obtained by dermal puncture than it is in blood obtained by venipuncture, and the concentrations of potassium, total protein, and calcium are lower. Therefore, alternating between dermal puncture and venipuncture should not be done when results for these analytes are to be compared, such as the glucose tolerance test. Note on the requisition form if the sample is from a dermal puncture.

TECHNICAL TIP 6-1

By documenting that the sample was collected by dermal puncture, the health-care provider can consider the collection technique when interpreting results.

DERMAL PUNCTURE EQUIPMENT

Dermal puncture supplies include automatic retractable safety puncture devices, microsample collection containers, 70 percent isopropyl alcohol pads, gauze pads, bandages, an approved sharps container, heel warmers, marking pen, glass slides, and gloves. With the exception of puncture devices, collection containers, heel warmers, and glass slides, the same equipment also is used for venipuncture.

Skin Puncture Devices

A variety of skin puncture devices are available in varying lengths and depths (see Fig. 6-1). All devices must have Occupational Safety & Health Administration (OSHA) required safety devices, such as retractable blades, to avoid possible exposure to bloodborne pathogens.

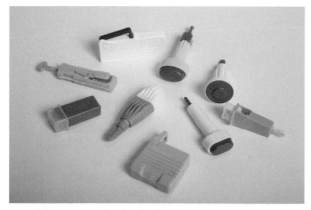

FIGURE 6-1 Dermal Puncture Devices. *(Reproduced with permission from Strasinger, S.K., and Di Lorenzo, M.S.: The Phlebotomy Textbook, ed. 3. Philadelphia, F.A. Davis, 2011.)*

To prevent contact with bone, the depth of the puncture produced by a device is critical. The incision depth of a skin puncture should be 2.0 to 2.5 mm for adults and should not exceed 2.0 mm for infants and small children. Manufacturers provide separate devices designed for heel punctures on premature infants, newborns, and babies and finger punctures on children and adults. The length of the lancets and the spring release mechanisms control the puncture depth with automatic devices. Punctures should never be performed using a surgical blade.

To produce adequate blood flow, the depth of the puncture is actually less important than the width of the puncture. As shown in **Figure 6-2,** the major vascular area of the skin is located at the dermal–subcutaneous juncture. The depth of this juncture can range from 0.35 to 1.6 mm in newborns to 3.0 mm in a large adult. Designated puncture devices easily reach it. Therefore, the number of severed capillaries depends on the width of the incision. Sufficient blood flow should be obtained from incision widths no larger than 2.5 mm.

Color-coded lancets indicating the varying depths and widths to accommodate low, medium, and high blood flow requirements are available. The type of device selected depends on the age of the patient, the amount of blood sample required, the collection site, and the puncture depth. BD Microtainer Contact-Activated Lancets (Becton, Dickinson, Franklin Lakes, NJ) are available in a full range of blades for microhematocrit tubes and Microtainer blood collection tubes and needles to collect blood for single-drop glucose testing **(Fig. 6-3)**. The BD Microtainer Contact-Activated Lancet is designed to activate only when the blade or needle is positioned and pressed against the skin. The BD Quikheel Lancets are color-coded heel-puncture lancets made specifically for premature infants, newborns, and babies **(Fig. 6-4)**.

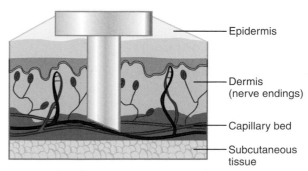

FIGURE 6-2 Vascular area of the skin. *(Reproduced with permission from Strasinger, S.K., and Di Lorenzo, M.S.: The Phlebotomy Textbook, ed. 3. Philadelphia, F.A. Davis, 2011.)*

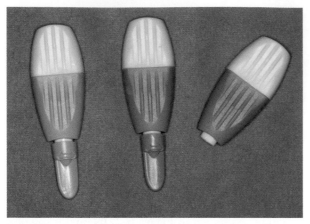

FIGURE 6-3 **BD Microtainer Contact-Activated Lancets.** *(Reproduced with permission from Strasinger, S.K., and Di Lorenzo, M.S.: The Phlebotomy Textbook, ed. 3. Philadelphia, F.A. Davis, 2011.)*

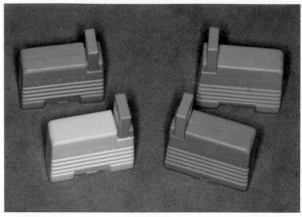

FIGURE 6-5 **Tenderfoot toddler (pink), newborn (pink/blue), preemie (white), and micropreemie (blue) heel incision devices (ITC, Edison, NJ).** *(Reproduced with permission from Strasinger, S.K., and Di Lorenzo, M.S.: The Phlebotomy Textbook, ed. 3. Philadelphia, F.A. Davis, 2011.)*

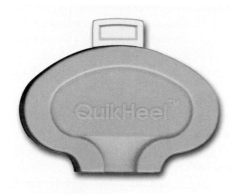

FIGURE 6-4 **Quikheel lancet.** *(Courtesy of Becton, Dickinson, Franklin Lakes, NJ.)*

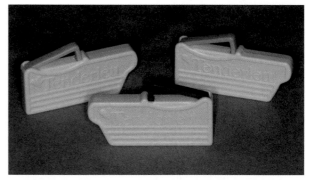

FIGURE 6-6 **Tenderlett Toddler, Junior, and Adult lancets (ITC, Edison, NJ).** *(Reproduced with permission from Strasinger, S.K., and Di Lorenzo, M.S.: The Phlebotomy Textbook, ed. 3. Philadelphia, F.A. Davis, 2011.)*

International Technidyne Corporation (Edison, NJ) produces a range of color-coded fully automated, single-use, retractable, disposable devices in varying depths. Tenderfoot and Tenderlett devices are designed for heel and finger punctures, respectively. Models are available ranging from the Tenderfoot for preemies **(Fig. 6-5)** to the Tenderlett for adults **(Fig. 6-6).**

Microsample Containers

Figure 6-7 illustrates some of the major sample containers available for collection of microsamples, including capillary tubes, micropipettes, and microcollection tubes. Some containers are designated for a specific test, and others serve multiple purposes.

Capillary Tubes

Capillary tubes, frequently referred to as microhematocrit tubes, are small plastic tubes that fill by capillary action

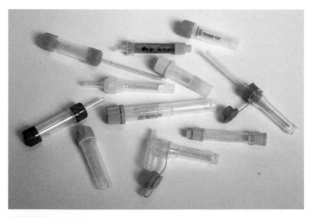

FIGURE 6-7 **Microsample containers.** *(Reproduced with permission from Strasinger, S.K., and Di Lorenzo, M.S.: The Phlebotomy Textbook, ed. 3. Philadelphia, F.A. Davis, 2011.)*

and are used to collect approximately 50 to 75 μL of blood for the primary purpose of performing a microhematocrit. The tubes are designed to fit into a hematocrit centrifuge and its corresponding hematocrit reader. Tubes are available plain or coated with ammonium heparin and are color-coded with a red band for heparinized tubes and a blue band for plain tubes. Heparinized tubes should be used for hematocrits collected by dermal puncture, and plain tubes are used when the test is being performed on previously anticoagulated blood. When sufficient blood has been collected, the end of the capillary tube that has not been used to collect the sample is closed with a clay sealant or a plastic plug. Tubes protected by plastic sleeves and self-sealing tubes are available to prevent breakage when collecting samples and sealing the microhematocrit tubes **(Fig. 6-8)**.

Micropipettes designed for capillary blood gas samples are available.

Microcollection Tubes

Plastic collection tubes such as the BD Microtainer Tube (Becton, Dickinson, Franklin Lakes, NJ) provide a larger collection volume. A variety of anticoagulants and additives, including separator gel, are available, and the tubes are color-coded in the same way as evacuated tubes. Amber-colored PST and SST Microtainers are available for light-sensitive analyte testing. Some tubes are supplied with a scoop collector top that is replaced by a color-coded

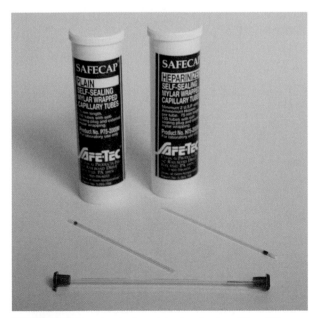

FIGURE 6-8 *(Reproduced with permission from Strasinger, S.K., and Di Lorenzo, M.S.: The Phlebotomy Textbook, ed. 3. Philadelphia, F.A. Davis, 2011.)*

plastic sealer top after the sample is collected. Microtainer tubes are designed to hold approximately 600 μL of blood.

BD Microtainer tubes with BD Microguard closures are designed to reduce the risk of blood splatter and blood leakage. The Microguard closure is removed by twisting and lifting. Tubes have a wide diameter, textured interior, and an integrated blood collection scoop to enhance blood flow into the tube and eliminate the need to assemble the equipment. After completion of the collection of blood, the cap is placed on the container, and anticoagulated tubes are gently inverted 5 to 10 times to ensure complete mixing. Tubes have markings to indicate minimum and maximum collection amounts to prevent underfilling or overfilling that could cause erroneous results. Tube extenders are available for this system to facilitate labeling and handling **(see Fig. 6-7)**. Separation of serum or plasma is achieved by centrifugation in specifically designed centrifuges.

Other capillary blood collection devices have plastic capillary tubes inserted into the collection container (SAFE-T-FILL capillary blood collection system, RAM Scientific Co., Needham, MA). After blood has been collected, the capillary tube is removed and the appropriate color-coded cap closes the tube.

DERMAL PUNCTURE PROCEDURE

Many of the procedures associated with venipuncture also apply to dermal puncture; therefore, the major emphasis in this chapter is on the techniques and complications that are unique to dermal puncture.

Blood Collector Preparation

The requisition form provides the information about the age of the patient and the test requested. This determines which of the variety of puncture devices and collection containers should be used for the dermal puncture. Patient identification may require confirmation from a parent or guardian. When a sample is collected by dermal puncture, it must be noted on the requisition form, because, as mentioned previously, the concentration of some analytes differs in venous and capillary blood.

 TECHNICAL TIP 6-2

Consider giving the parents the option to stay with the child or leave the room.

Patient Preparation

For optimal blood flow, the area to be punctured may be warmed. This is primarily a concern for patients with very cold or cyanotic fingers, for heel punctures to collect multiple samples, and for the collection of capillary blood gases. Warming dilates the blood vessels and increases arterial blood flow. Warming is performed by moistening a towel with warm water (42°C) or by activating a commercial heel warmer and covering the site for 3 to 5 minutes (Fig. 6-9).

Patient Position

The patient must be seated or lying down with the hand supported on a firm surface, palm up, and fingers pointed downward for finger punctures. For heel punctures, infants should be lying on the back with the heel in a downward position.

Site Selection

The choice of a puncture area is based on the age and size of the patient. Select puncture sites that provide sufficient distance between the skin and the bone to avoid accidental contact with the bone that may cause infection (osteomyelitis). The primary sites are the heel and the distal segments of the third and fourth fingers. Performing dermal punctures on earlobes is usually not recommended.

Areas selected for dermal puncture should not be calloused, scarred, bruised, edematous, cold or cyanotic, or infected. Punctures should never be made through previous puncture sites, because this can easily introduce microorganisms into the puncture and allow them to reach the bone. Do not collect blood from the fingers on the side of a mastectomy without a health-care provider's order.

Heel Puncture Sites

The heel is the most common site for dermal punctures on infants younger than 1 year of age because it contains more tissue than the fingers and has not yet become calloused from walking. Acceptable areas for heel puncture are shown in **Figure 6-10** and are described as the medial and lateral areas of the bottom (plantar) surface of the heel. These areas can be determined by drawing imaginary lines extending back from the middle of the large toe and from between the fourth and fifth toes. It is in these areas that the distance between the skin and the heel bone (calcaneus) is greatest. Notice the short distance between the back (posterior curvature) of the heel and the calcaneus. This is the reason that this area is never acceptable for heel puncture.

Punctures should not be performed in other areas of the foot, and particularly not in the arch, where they may cause damage to nerves and tendons.

Heel Puncture Sites

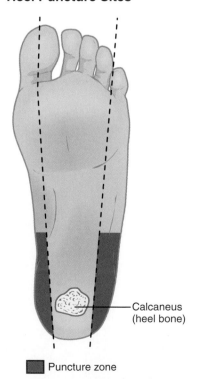

Calcaneus
(heel bone)

▮ Puncture zone

FIGURE 6-10 Acceptable heel puncture sites. *(Reproduced with permission from Strasinger, S.K., and Di Lorenzo, M.S.: The Phlebotomy Textbook, ed. 3. Philadelphia, F.A. Davis, 2011.)*

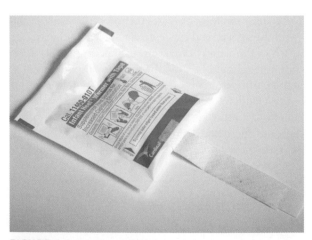

FIGURE 6-9 Commercial heel warmer. *(Reproduced with permission from Strasinger, S.K., and Di Lorenzo, M.S.: The Phlebotomy Textbook, ed. 3. Philadelphia, F.A. Davis, 2011.)*

Finger Puncture Sites

Finger punctures are performed on adults and children older than 1 year of age. Fingers of infants younger than 1 year old may not contain enough tissue to prevent contact with the bone and require a heel puncture.

The fleshy areas located near the center of the third and fourth fingers on the **palmar** side are the sites of choice for finger puncture **(Fig. 6-11).** Because the tip and sides of the finger contain only about half the tissue mass of the central area, the possibility of bone injury is increased in these areas. Problems associated with the use of other fingers include possible callouses on the thumb, increased nerve endings in the index finger, and decreased tissue in the fifth finger **(Box 6-1).**

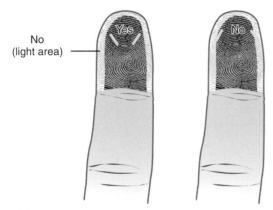

No (light area)

Yes   No

FIGURE 6-11 Acceptable finger puncture sites and correct puncture angle. *(Reproduced with permission from Strasinger, S.K., and Di Lorenzo, M.S.: The Phlebotomy Textbook, ed. 3. Philadelphia, F.A. Davis, 2011.)*

BOX 6-1 Summary of Dermal Puncture Site Selection

- Use the medial and lateral areas of the plantar surface of the heel.
- Use the central fleshy area of the third or fourth fingers.
- Do not use the fingers on the side of a mastectomy.
- Do not use the back of the heel.
- Do not use the arch of the foot.
- Do not puncture through old sites.
- Do not use areas with visible damage.
- Do not use fingers on newborns or children younger than 1 year.
- Do not use swollen sites.
- Do not use earlobes.

Cleansing the Site

The selected site is cleansed with 70 percent isopropyl alcohol using a circular motion. The alcohol should be allowed to dry on the skin for maximum bacteriostatic action, and the residue removed with gauze to prevent possible interference with test results. Failure to allow the alcohol to dry will:

1. Cause a stinging sensation for the patient
2. Contaminate the sample
3. Hemolyze RBCs
4. Prevent formation of a rounded blood drop because blood will mix with the alcohol and run down the finger

 TECHNICAL TIP 6-3

Use of povidone-iodine is not recommended for dermal punctures because sample contamination may elevate some test results, including bilirubin, phosphorus, uric acid, and potassium.

Performing the Puncture

While the puncture is performed, the heel or finger should be well supported and held firmly, without squeezing the puncture area. Massaging the area before the puncture may increase blood flow to the area.

Heel Puncture

The heel is held between the thumb and index finger of the nondominant hand with the index finger held over the heel and the thumb below the heel.

Finger Puncture

The finger is held between the nondominant thumb and index finger, with the palmar surface facing up and the finger pointing downward to increase blood flow.

Puncture Device Position

Place the puncture device firmly on the puncture site. Do not indent the skin when placing the lancet on the puncture site. The blade of the lancet should be aligned to cut across (perpendicular to) the grooves of the finger or heel print. This prevents the blood from running into the grooves that prevent the formation of a rounded drop of blood.

Activate the lancet and hold for a moment, then release. Pressure must be maintained, because the elasticity of the skin naturally inhibits penetration of the blade. Removal of the lancet before the puncture is complete will yield a low blood flow.

TECHNICAL TIP 6-4

Failure to place puncture devices firmly on the skin is the primary cause of insufficient blood flow. One firm puncture is less painful for the patient than two "mini" punctures.

Puncture Device Disposal

After completing the puncture, the puncture device should be placed in an approved sharps container. A new puncture device must be used if an additional puncture is required.

Sample Collection

Microhematocrit Tubes and Micropipettes

Before beginning the collection, wipe away the first drop of blood with gauze. This will prevent contamination of the sample with residual alcohol and tissue fluid released during the puncture. When collecting microsamples, even a minute amount of contamination can severely affect the sample quality. Therefore, blood should be flowing freely from the puncture site as a result of firm pressure and should not be obtained by milking or strenuous massaging of the surrounding tissue that will release tissue fluid. The most satisfactory blood flow is obtained by alternately applying and releasing pressure to the area. Tightly squeezing the area with no relaxation will cut off blood flow to the puncture site.

TECHNICAL TIP 6-5

Applying pressure about ½ inch away from the puncture site frequently produces better blood flow than pressure very close to the site.

TECHNICAL TIP 6-6

Some point-of-care instruments do not require that the first drop of blood be wiped away. Always follow the manufacturer's instructions.

Because microhematocrit tubes fill by capillary action, the collection tip can be lightly touched to the drop of blood and the blood will be drawn into the tube. Fingers are positioned slightly downward with the palmar surface also facing slightly down during the collection procedure. To prevent introduction of air bubbles, capillary tubes and micropipettes are held horizontally while being filled. The presence of air bubbles limits the amount of blood that can be collected per tube and interferes with blood gas determinations. When the tubes are filled, they are sealed with sealant clay or designated plastic caps.

TECHNICAL TIP 6-7

While collecting the sample, the patient's hand does not have to be completely turned over. Rotating the hand 90 degrees allows blood collectors to clearly see the blood drops without placing themselves in awkward positions.

Microcollection Containers

Microcollection containers are slanted down during the collection, and blood is allowed to run through the collection scoop and down the side of the tube. The tip of the collection container is placed beneath the puncture site and touches the underside of the drop. The first three drops of blood provide the channel to allow blood to flow freely into the container. Gently tapping the bottom of the tube may be necessary to force blood to the bottom. Collection devices should not touch the puncture site and should not be scraped over the skin, because this will produce sample contamination and hemolysis. When a tube is filled, the color-coded top is attached. Tubes with anticoagulants should be inverted 5 to 10 times. If blood flow is slow, it may be necessary to mix the tube while the collection is in progress. It is important to work quickly, because blood that takes more than 2 minutes to collect may form microclots in an anticoagulated microcollection container.

TECHNICAL TIP 6-8

Strong consistent squeezing (milking) must be avoided because it can cause hemolysis or tissue-fluid contamination of the sample.

TECHNICAL TIP 6-9

Using a scooping motion to collect the blood must be avoided because it can hemolyze the sample.

TECHNICAL TIP 6-10

Fast collection and mixing ensure more accurate test results.

Order of Collection

The order of draw for collecting multiple samples from a dermal puncture is different from venipuncture because of the tendency of platelets to accumulate at the site of a wound. Blood to be used for tests for the evaluation of platelets, such as blood smear, platelet count, and complete blood count (CBC), must be collected first. The blood smear should be made first, followed by the lavender ethylenediaminetetraacetic acid (EDTA) microcollection container. The following is the order of collection for multiple tubes:

- Capillary blood gases
- Blood smear
- EDTA microcollection container
- Other anticoagulated microcollection containers
- Serum microcollection container

Bandaging the Patient

When sufficient blood has been collected, pressure is applied to the puncture site with gauze. The finger or heel is elevated and pressure is applied until the bleeding stops. Confirm that the bleeding has stopped before removing the pressure.

Bandages are not used for children younger than 2 years of age because they may remove the bandages,

place them in the mouth, and possibly aspirate the bandages. The adhesive may also cause irritation to sensitive skin, particularly the fragile skin of a newborn or older adult patient.

Labeling the Sample

Microsamples must be labeled with the same information required for venipuncture samples. Labels can be wrapped around microcollection tubes or groups of microhematocrit tubes. For transport, microhematocrit tubes are then placed in a large tube, because the outside of the microhematocrit tubes may be contaminated with blood and to prevent breakage.

Becton, Dickinson Microtainer collection tubes have extenders that can be attached to the container. This allows the computer label to be applied vertically.

Completion of the Procedure

The dermal puncture procedure is completed by disposing of all used materials in appropriate containers, removing gloves, sanitizing hands, and thanking the patient and/or the parents for their cooperation.

All special handling procedures associated with venipuncture samples also apply to microsamples. Observe test collection priorities.

To prevent excessive removal of blood from small infants, a log sheet for documenting the amount of blood collected each time a procedure is requested may be required by facility policy.

As with venipuncture, it is recommended that only two punctures be attempted to collect the blood. When a second puncture must be made to collect the sufficient amount of blood, the blood should not be added to the previously collected tube. This can cause erroneous results because of microclots and hemolysis.

TECHNICAL TIP 6-11

Clotting is triggered immediately on skin puncture and represents the greatest obstacle in collecting quality samples.

Procedure 6-1 describes the technique unique to the finger puncture and **Procedure 6-2** shows the heel puncture technique.

PROCEDURE 6-1 Collection of Blood From a Finger Puncture

EQUIPMENT:

Gloves
70 percent isopropyl alcohol pad
Finger puncture device
Microcollection container

Gauze
Warming device
Sharps container
Indelible pen

PROCEDURE:

Step 1. Obtain and examine the requisition form.

Step 2. Greet the patient, explain the procedure to be performed, and obtain informed consent.

Step 3. Identify the patient verbally by having him or her state both the first name and last name and compare the information on the patient's ID band with the requisition form. A parent or guardian may do this for a child.

Step 4. Prepare the patient and/or parents and verify diet restrictions, as appropriate, allergies to latex, or previous problems with blood collection.

Step 5. Position the patient's arm on a firm surface with the hand palm up. The child may have to be held in either the vertical or horizontal restraint.

Step 6. Select equipment according to the age of patient, the type of test ordered, and the amount of blood to be collected.

Step 7. Sanitize hands and put on gloves.

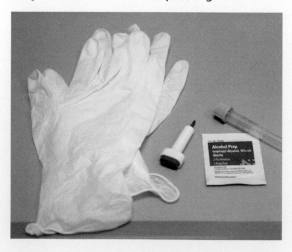

Step 8. Select the puncture site in the fleshy areas located off the center of the third or fourth fingers on the palmar side of the nondominant hand. Do not use the side or tip of the finger.

Step 9. Warm the puncture site if necessary.

Step 10. Cleanse and dry the puncture site with 70 percent isopropyl alcohol in concentric circles and allow to air-dry.

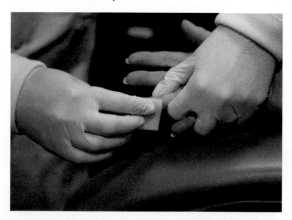

Step 11. Prepare the lancet by removing the lancet locking device and open the cap to the microcollection container.

Step 12. Hold the finger between the nondominant thumb and index finger, with the palmar surface facing up and the finger pointing downward.

PROCEDURE 6-1 Collection of Blood From a Finger Puncture (Continued)

Step 13. Place the lancet firmly on the fleshy area of the finger perpendicular to the fingerprint and depress the lancet trigger.

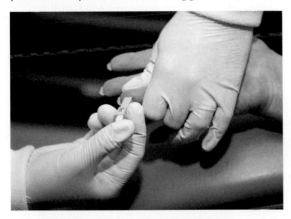

Step 14. Discard lancet in the approved sharps container.

Step 15. Gently squeeze the finger and wipe away the first drop of blood that may contain alcohol residue and tissue fluid.

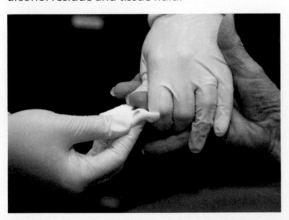

Step 16. Collect rounded drops into microcollection containers in the correct order of draw without scraping the skin. Do not milk the site. Collect the sample within 2 minutes to prevent clotting

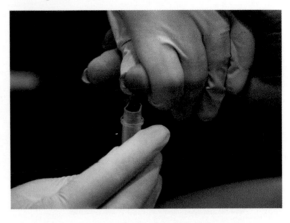

Step 17. Cap the microcollection container when the correct amount of blood has been collected.

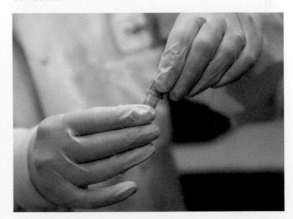

PROCEDURE 6-1 **Collection of Blood From a Finger Puncture** (Continued)

Step 18. Mix microcollection containers 5 to 10 times by gentle inversion as recommended by the manufacturer. They may have to be gently tapped throughout the procedure to mix the blood with the anticoagulant.

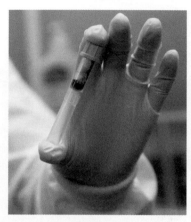

Step 20. Label the microcollection containers before leaving the patient and verify identification with the patient ID band or verbally with an outpatient. Observe any special handling procedures.

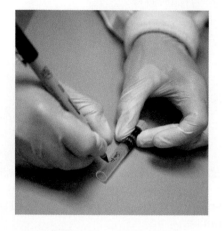

Step 19. Place gauze on the site and ask the patient or parent to apply pressure until bleeding stops.

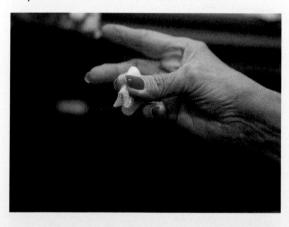

Step 21. Examine the site for stoppage of bleeding and apply bandage if the patient is older than 2 years.

Step 22. Dispose of used supplies in biohazard containers.

Step 23. Thank the patient.

Step 24. Remove gloves and sanitize hands.

Step 25. Complete requisition form.

Step 26. Prepare sample for transportation to the laboratory.

Reproduced with permission from Strasinger, S.K., and Di Lorenzo, M.S.: The Phlebotomy Textbook, ed. 3. Philadelphia, F.A. Davis, 2011.

PROCEDURE 6-2 Collection of Blood by Heel Puncture

EQUIPMENT:

Gloves	Gauze
70 percent isopropyl alcohol pad	Warming device
Heel puncture device	Sharps container
Microcollection container	Indelible pen

PROCEDURE:

Step 1. Obtain and examine the requisition form.

Step 2. Place collection tray in a designated area.

Step 3. Check requisition form and select necessary equipment.

Step 4. Sanitize hands and put on gloves. Put on a gown if it is a nursery requirement.

Step 5. Identify patient by comparing the ID band that is attached to the baby with the requisition form.

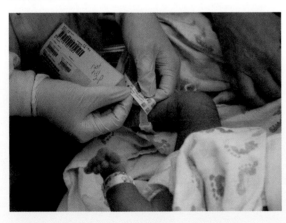

Step 6. Position the baby lying on his or her back with the foot lower than the body.

Step 7. Warm the heel for 3 to 5 minutes by wrapping the heel with a warm washcloth or using a commercial heel-warming device.

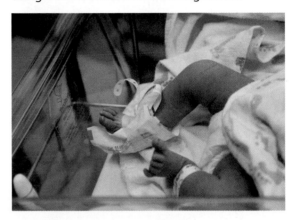

Step 8. Select the puncture site on the medial or lateral plantar surface of the heel. Do not use the arch or back of the heel.

Step 9. Cleanse the puncture site with 70 percent isopropyl alcohol and allow it to air-dry.

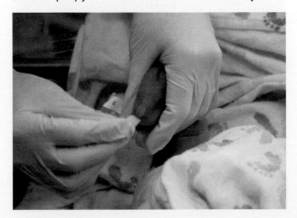

PROCEDURE 6-2 Collection of Blood by Heel Puncture (Continued)

Step 10. Prepare the lancet by removing the lancet locking device and open the cap to the microcollection container.

Step 11. Hold the heel firmly by wrapping the heel with the nondominant hand.

Step 12. Place the lancet perpendicular to the heel print and depress the lancet trigger.

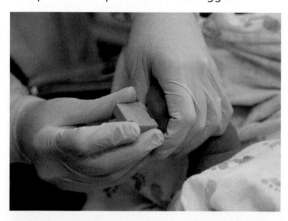

Step 13. Discard the lancet in an approved sharps container.

Step 14. Wipe away the first drop of blood.

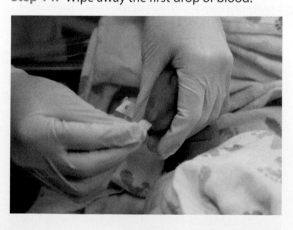

Step 15. Collect rounded drops of blood into microcollection containers without scraping the skin. Do not milk the site.

Step 16. Collect the proper amount of blood in the correct order of draw.

Step 17. Mix microcollection containers 5 to 10 times and/or seal microhematocrit tubes.

Step 18. Place gauze on site and apply pressure until bleeding stops.

Step 19. Label tubes and observe any special handling procedures.

Step 20. Check the site for bleeding. Do not place a bandage on an infant younger than 2 years.

Step 21. Dispose of used supplies and remove all collection equipment from the area.

Step 22. Remove gloves (and gown if wearing one) and sanitize hands.

Step 23. Complete patient log sheet.

Step 24. Prepare sample and requisition for transportation to the laboratory.

Reproduced with permission from Strasinger, S.K., and Di Lorenzo, M.S.: The Phlebotomy Textbook, ed. 3. Philadelphia, F.A. Davis, 2011.

SPECIAL DERMAL COLLECTIONS

Collection of Newborn Bilirubin

One of the most frequently performed tests on newborns measures bilirubin levels, and samples for this determination are often collected at timed intervals over several days. Bilirubin is a very light-sensitive substance and is rapidly destroyed when exposed to light.

Blood collection technique is critical to the determination of accurate bilirubin results, and samples must be collected quickly and protected from excess light during and after the collection. Infants who appear **jaundiced** are frequently placed under an ultraviolet light (UV) to lower the level of circulating bilirubin. This light must be turned off during sample collection. Amber-colored microcollection tubes are available for collecting bilirubin, or if multiple capillary pipettes are used, the filled tubes should be shielded from light. Hemolysis must be avoided; it will falsely lower bilirubin results in some procedures and must be corrected for in others. Samples must be collected at the specified time so that the rate of bilirubin increase can be determined.

 TECHNICAL TIP 6-12

Be sure to turn off the ultraviolet light when collecting samples for neonatal bilirubin tests.

 TECHNICAL TIP 6-13

Bilirubin levels may decrease as much as 50 percent in a blood sample that has been exposed to light for 2 hours.

Collection of Newborn Screening Tests

Newborn screening is the testing of newborn babies for genetic, metabolic, hormonal, and functional disorders that can cause physical disabilities, mental retardation, or even death, if not detected and treated early. Screening of newborns for 50 inherited metabolic disorders can currently be performed from blood collected by heel puncture and placed on specially designed filter paper. Each state has its own laws requiring specific screening of newborns; however, all states screen newborns for the presence of the

most prevalent disorders. Examples of the common disorders phenylketonuria (PKU), congenital hypothyroidism, and galactosemia are described **Box 6-2.** Many of these disorders can be prevented by early changes in the newborns diet or early administration of a missing hormone.

Blood Collection

Newborn screening tests are performed on blood collected by dermal puncture, except for the hearing test. Blood is collected between 24 and 48 hours after birth, before the baby is released from the hospital. Correct collection of the blood sample is critical for accurate test results. The Clinical and Laboratory Standards Institute (CLSI) standards recommend that the newborn

---

BOX 6-2 Mandatory Newborn Screening Disorders

PHENYLKETONURIA

Phenylketonuria (PKU) is caused by the lack of the enzyme needed to metabolize the amino acid phenylalanine to tyrosine, which accumulates and causes problems with brain development and other delays in physical, mental and social skills. Early detection is crucial because the damage is irreversible but can be treated with a diet low in phenylalanine and high in tyrosine.

CONGENITAL HYPOTHYROIDISM

Congenital hypothyroidism is a thyroid hormone deficiency present at birth. Delays in growth and brain development that produce physical and developmental abnormalities can be avoided by the use of oral doses of thyroid hormone within the first few weeks after birth.

GALACTOSEMIA

Galactosemia is a genetic metabolic disorder caused by the lack of the liver enzyme needed to convert galactose (sugar in milk) into glucose. Galactose accumulates in the blood and can cause liver disease, renal failure, cataracts, blindness, mental retardation, and death. Treatment is the elimination of all milk and dairy products from the infant for life.

Reproduced with permission from Strasinger, S.K., and Di Lorenzo, M.S.: The Phlebotomy Textbook, ed. 3. Philadelphia, F.A. Davis, 2011.

screening samples should be collected separately, after prewarming and puncturing a second site when additional blood tests are requested.

Special collection kits are used, consisting of a patient information form attached to specifically designed filter paper that has been preprinted with an appropriate number of ½-inch-diameter circles that are part of the requisition form **(Fig. 6-12).** The blood collector must be careful not to touch or contaminate the area inside the circles or to touch the dried blood spots. Care must be taken to avoid contaminating the sample with water, formula, alcohol, urine, lotions, or powder.

The heel puncture is performed in the routine manner, and the first drop of blood is wiped away. A large drop of blood is then applied directly into a filter paper circle. Do not touch the filter paper to the heel. To obtain an even layer of blood, only one large free-falling drop should be used to fill a circle. Blood is applied to only one side of the filter paper, and there must be enough to soak through the paper and be visible on the other side. Each circle must be filled for testing. As shown in **Figure 6-13,** if a circle is not evenly or completely filled, a new circle and a larger drop of blood should be used. The collected sample must be allowed to air-dry in a suspended horizontal position, at room temperature, and away from direct sunlight. To prevent cross-contamination, samples should not be hung to dry or stacked during or after the drying process. After drying for at least 3 hours, the sample is

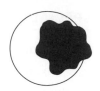

| Acceptable specimen | Uneven application of blood | Circle not completely filled |

FIGURE 6-13 **Correct and incorrect blood collection with filter paper.** *(Reproduced with permission from Strasinger, S.K., and Di Lorenzo, M.S.: The Phlebotomy Textbook, ed. 3. Philadelphia, F.A. Davis, 2011.)*

placed in a special envelope and sent to the appropriate laboratory for testing. **Procedure 6-3** describes the technique for collecting blood for newborn screening.

TECHNICAL TIP 6-14

Be sure that all required patient information is completely filled out on the newborn screening test form.

TECHNICAL TIP 6-15

Specific state mandates for newborn screening can be found at the U.S. National Newborn Screening and Genetics Resource Center website: http://genes-r-us.uthscsa.edu/

TECHNICAL TIP 6-16

Uneven or incomplete saturation of PKU filter paper circles because of layering from multidrop applications will yield an unacceptable sample for testing.

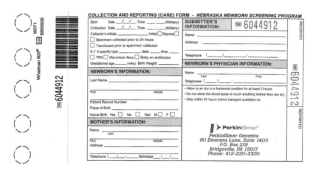

FIGURE 6-12 **Newborn screening sample form.** *(Reproduced with permission from Strasinger, S.K., and Di Lorenzo, M.S.: The Phlebotomy Textbook, ed. 3. Philadelphia, F.A. Davis, 2011.)*

PROCEDURE 6-3 Newborn Screening Blood Collection

EQUIPMENT:

Newborn screening filter paper form
Gloves
70 percent isopropyl alcohol pad
Heel puncture device

Gauze
Warming device
Sharps container
Indelible pen

PROCEDURE:

Step 1. Perform Steps 1 to 14 of Procedure 12-2: Collection of Blood by Heel Puncture.

Step 2. Touch the filter paper to a large drop of blood.

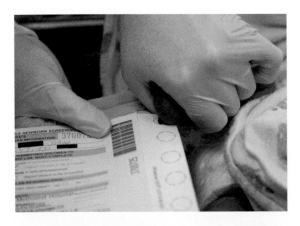

Step 3. Evenly fill the circle on one side of the filter paper, allowing the blood to soak through the paper to be visible on the other side.

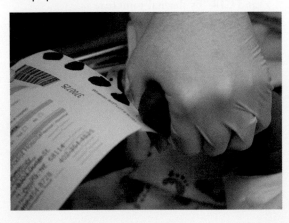

Step 4. Fill all required circles correctly.

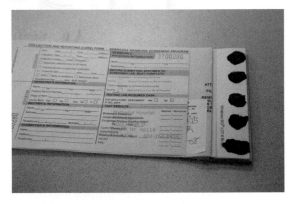

Step 5. Place gauze on site and apply pressure until bleeding stops.

Step 6. Place the filter paper in a suspended horizontal position to dry for a minimum of 3 hours. Do not stack multiple filter papers.

Step 7. Label the sample and place it in the special envelope when dry.

Step 8. Check the site for bleeding. Do not place a bandage on an infant.

Step 9. Dispose of used supplies and remove all collection equipment from the area.

Step 10. Remove gloves (and gown if wearing one) and sanitize hands.

Step 11. Complete patient log sheet.

Step 12. Prepare sample and requisition form for transportation to laboratory and for mailing to the reference testing agency.

Reproduced with permission from Strasinger, S.K., and Di Lorenzo, M.S.: The Phlebotomy Textbook, ed. 3. Philadelphia, F.A. Davis, 2011.

BIBLIOGRAPHY

CLSI: *Blood Collection on Filter Paper for Newborn Screening Programs; Approved Standard*, ed. 5. CLSI Document LA04-A5. Wayne, PA, CLSI, 2007.

CLSI: *Procedures and Devices for the Collection of Diagnostic Capillary Blood Specimens; Approved Standard*, ed. 6. CLSI document GP42-A6 (H04-A6). Wayne, PA, CLSI, 2009.

March of Dimes: Recommended Newborn Screening Tests: 29 Disorders. http://www.marchofdimes.com/professionals/14332_15455.asp.

Strasinger, S.K., and DiLorenzo, M.S.: *The Phlebotomy Textbook*, ed. 3. Philadelphia, FA Davis, 2011.

INTERNET RESOURCES

www.bd.com

www.clsi.org

www.itcmed.com

www.cellrobotics.com

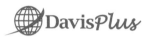 For additional material, please visit http://davisplus.fadavis.com.

REVIEW QUESTIONS

1. When selecting a dermal puncture device, the most critical consideration is the:
   a. Width of the incision
   b. Amount of blood needed
   c. Depth of the incision
   d. Test requested

2. Why should a dermal collection site be warmed?
   a. Prevents hemolysis
   b. Increases blood flow
   c. Prevents clotting
   d. Causes hemoconcentration

3. Capillary punctures on newborns are performed on the:
   a. Index finger
   b. Plantar area of the heel
   c. Back of the heel
   d. Earlobe

4. Failure to allow the alcohol to dry on the puncture site may cause:
   a. Inability to form a rounded drop
   b. Sample contamination
   c. Red blood cell hemolysis
   d. All of the above

5. Wiping away the first drop of blood:
   a. Increases blood flow
   b. Prevents sample contamination
   c. Causes air bubbles to enter the tube
   d. Stimulates platelets and faster clotting

6. The possibility of infection is increased when:
   a. The thumb is punctured
   b. Alcohol is used to cleanse the site
   c. A puncture is made through a previous site
   d. The palmar side of the finger is punctured

7. Failure to puncture across the fingerprint during a finger puncture will cause:
   a. Blood to run down the finger
   b. Hemolysis
   c. Contamination of the sample
   d. Additional patient discomfort

8. Selection of an improper heel puncture site can result in:
   a. Puncture of the calcaneous
   b. Sample hemolysis
   c. The need for vigorous massaging
   d. Increased blood flow

9. The order of draw for a bilirubin, blood smear, and CBC by dermal puncture is:
   a. CBC, blood smear, and bilirubin
   b. Blood smear, CBC, and bilirubin
   c. Bilirubin, blood smear, and CBC
   d. Blood smear, bilirubin, and CBC

10. A test included in a newborn screen is:
    a. PKU
    b. Electrolytes
    c. Bilirubin
    d. CBC

FOR FURTHER STUDY

1. State a major concern when collecting a sample for potassium and bilirubin by dermal puncture.

2. Can dermal puncture and venipuncture collections be alternated on a patient when collecting samples for a glucose tolerance test? Why or why not?

3. Explain why a sample for a bilirubin test that has been sitting on the counter for 3 hours would be rejected.

4. Name two causes of osteomyelitis associated with dermal puncture.

CASE STUDY 6-1

Sharon, the laboratory manager, notices that many of the blood samples collected at the pediatric office are hemolyzed. Sharon suggests a continuing education in-service class for the clinic.

1. Why should preparation of the collection site be stressed?

2. Why is it important for the personnel to obtain rounded drops of blood to prevent hemolysis?

3. Should the in-service class include the procedure to follow when a second puncture must be performed to obtain a full tube of blood? Why or why not?

CASE STUDY 6-2

Lisa, the medical assistant, collects a lavender top Microtainer and a red top Microtainer by dermal puncture from a newborn's heel in the physician's office. The doctor is concerned because the platelet count is much lower than the previous day's result when the blood was tested before the newborn was released from the hospital. All other CBC parameters match the previous values. The serum in the red top Microtainer appears hemolyzed.

1. Could the blood collection technique have caused this?

2. Why or why not?

3. What factors could cause hemolysis in the tubes?

EVALUATION OF A FINGER PUNCTURE FOR A MICROHEMATOCRIT

RATING SYSTEM

2 = Satisfactory

1 = Needs improvement

0 = Incorrect/did not perform

_____ 1. Greets patient, explains procedure, and obtains informed consent.

_____ 2. Examines requisition form.

_____ 3. Asks patient to state full name and date of birth.

_____ 4. Compares requisition information and patient's statement.

_____ 5. Compares requisition information with ID band.

_____ 6. Sanitizes hands and puts on gloves.

_____ 7. Organizes and assembles equipment.

_____ 8. Selects appropriate finger.

_____ 9. Warms finger, if necessary.

_____ 10. Gently massages finger.

_____ 11. Cleanses site with 70 percent alcohol and allows it to air-dry.

_____ 12. Removes lancet locking device and does not contaminate puncture device.

_____ 13. Smoothly performs puncture across fingerprint.

_____ 14. Disposes of puncture device in sharps container.

_____ 15. Wipes away first drop of blood.

_____ 16. Collects two microhematocrit tubes without air bubbles.

_____ 17. Seals tubes.

_____ 18. Applies gauze to site and asks patient to apply pressure.

_____ 19. Labels tubes and confirms the information with the ID band or patient.

_____ 20. Examines site for stoppage of bleeding and applies bandage.

_____ 21. Disposes of used supplies.

_____ 22. Removes gloves.

_____ 23. Sanitizes hands.

_____ 24. Thanks patient.

TOTAL POINTS

MAXIMUM POINTS = 48

COMMENTS:

EVALUATION OF A MICROTAINER COLLECTION BY HEEL PUNCTURE

RATING SYSTEM

2 = Satisfactory

1 = Needs improvement

0 = Incorrect/did not perform

_____ 1. Places collection tray in designated area.

_____ 2. Examines requisition form.

_____ 3. Sanitizes hands and puts on gloves.

_____ 4. Organizes and assembles equipment.

_____ 5. Identifies patient using ID band.

_____ 6. Warms heel.

_____ 7. Selects appropriate puncture site.

_____ 8. Cleanses puncture site with 70 percent alcohol and allows it to air-dry.

_____ 9. Removes lancet locking device and does not contaminate puncture device.

_____ 10. Performs puncture smoothly across the heel print.

_____ 11. Disposes of puncture device in sharps container.

_____ 12. Wipes away first drop of blood.

_____ 13. Collects rounded drops into microcollection container without scraping.

_____ 14. Does not milk site.

_____ 15. Collects adequate amount of blood.

_____ 16. Mixes microcollection container 5 to 10 times.

_____ 17. Cleanses site and applies pressure until bleeding stops.

_____ 18. Removes all collection equipment from area.

_____ 19. Disposes of used supplies.

_____ 20. Labels tube and verifies identification.

_____ 21. Removes and disposes of gloves.

_____ 22. Sanitizes hands.

_____ 23. Completes patient blood collection log sheet.

TOTAL POINTS

MAXIMUM POINTS = 46

COMMENTS:

EVALUATION OF NEONATAL FILTER PAPER COLLECTION

RATING SYSTEM

2 = Satisfactory

1 = Needs Improvement

0 = Incorrect/Did Not Perform

_____ 1. Examines requisition form.

_____ 2. Sanitizes hands and puts on gloves.

_____ 3. Identifies patient using the ID band.

_____ 4. Organizes and assembles equipment.

_____ 5. Selects appropriate heel site.

_____ 6. Warms heel.

_____ 7. Cleanses site with 70 percent alcohol and allows it to air-dry.

_____ 8. Removes lancet locking device and does not contaminate puncture device.

_____ 9. Performs the puncture across the heel print.

_____ 10. Wipes away first blood drop.

_____ 11. Evenly fills a circle.

_____ 12. Fills all required circles correctly.

_____ 13. Does not touch inside of circles or blood spots.

_____ 14. Places filter paper in appropriate transport position.

_____ 15. Applies pressure until bleeding stops.

_____ 16. Disposes of equipment and supplies.

_____ 17. Correctly completes all required paperwork.

_____ 18. Removes gloves.

_____ 19. Sanitizes hands.

_____ 20. Delivers sample to laboratory for mailing to reference testing agency.

TOTAL POINTS

MAXIMUM POINTS = 40

COMMENTS:

Point-of-Care Testing

Upon completion of this chapter, the reader will be able to:

7.1 Define point-of-care testing (POCT).

7.2 List tests performed at the point of care (POC).

7.3 Identify the three phases of laboratory testing.

7.4 Explain the POCT quality control procedures for Clinical Laboratory Improvements Amendments (CLIA) compliance.

7.5 Discuss critical elements for POCTs.

7.6 Discuss CLIA complexity, competency testing, quality management, and regulatory requirements.

KEY TERMS

Calibration Standardization of an instrument used to perform diagnostic tests

Critical Value Laboratory test result critical to patient survival

Point-of-Care Testing Laboratory tests performed in the patient care area

Proficiency Testing Performance of tests on specimens provided by an external monitoring agency

Quality Control Methods used to monitor the accuracy of procedures

Quality Management Methods used to guarantee quality patient care

Reference Range Laboratory test results that are within normal limits

INTRODUCTION

Point-of-care testing (POCT) is laboratory testing performed at or near the patient bedside. POCT also may be referred to as "near patient testing," "bedside testing," POCT, or POC. Although POCT is laboratory testing, the majority of POCT is performed by nonlaboratory personnel. POCT personnel, also referred to as "operators," are usually primary patient care providers. This group of operators includes nurses, respiratory therapists, physicians, laboratory, medical, and nursing assistants, phlebotomists, and other health-care professionals. POCT is used in many patient care settings including emergency departments, intensive care units, surgical suites, radiology units, physician office clinics, health fairs, dialysis units, and other health-care settings.

As technology has advanced, the scope of POCT and its role in providing quality patient care has expanded at an exponential rate. **Table 7-1** lists commonly performed POCTs and their associated laboratory section.

Manufacturers have continued to expand the list of available POCTs and the sample types that can be analyzed. Whole blood, urine, and direct swabs from an infected area are still the most common sample types, but saliva, breath, and other body fluids also are being used. Some newer technologies do not require a sample, such as the devices that perform transcutaneous bilirubin, oximetry, and noninvasive glucose testing. These technologies are capable of obtaining a laboratory answer by placing the POCT device directly on the patient's skin without obtaining a sample from the patient.

The rapid growth of POCT technology has provided health-care professionals the mobility to bring a large test menu of rapid laboratory services to the patient's

TABLE 7-1 Common POCTs Associated with Laboratory Departments

Laboratory Department	Tests
Hematology	Hemoglobin Hematocrit Erythrocyte sedimentation rate (ESR) White blood cell count (WBC)
Chemistry	Glucose, arterial blood gases (ABGs), lipid panel, blood urea nitrogen (BUN), creatinine, electrolytes, comprehensive metabolic profile, cardiac markers, liver function tests, human chorionic gonadotropin (HCG), hemoglobin A_{1c}
Serology	HIV, infectious mononucleosis, *Helicobacter pylori*, HCG
Urinalysis and body fluids	Reagent strip urinalysis, occult blood, body fluid pH
Urine toxicology (drugs of abuse)	Amphetamines, marijuana, cocaine, benzodiazepines, barbiturates, ethanol
Microbiology	Group A *Streptococcus*, influenza A/B, respiratory syncytial virus (RSV), bacterial vaginosis (BV)
Coagulation	Prothrombin time (PT)/international normalizing ratio (INR), activated partial thromboplastin time (APTT), activated clotting time (ACT)

bedside. Other advantages to POCT may include decreased turnaround time (TAT) for test results, decreased sample volume, reduction or elimination of sample transport to the main laboratory, simple testing procedure (ease of use), decreased analyzer size, and increased opportunity for more personal patient interaction with nursing or other designated care providers.

POCT also has several identified drawbacks. Because POCT is true laboratory testing, it also is governed by all of the same regulations that apply to laboratory testing performed in a traditional laboratory. Accreditation requirements, charging and billing mechanisms, documentation of patient results, **quality control** (QC) testing and documentation, intended use, cost, and inventory management are all processes that can be problematic. In many settings, a large number of patient care providers perform POCTs compared with a much smaller number of laboratory staff who would be performing the test in a traditional laboratory setting. The large number of operators can have a dilution effect on operator competency. This is particularly apparent when the volume of POCTs is low and the number of operators is high. The operators have fewer opportunities to maintain their skill level, because the test is performed at a very low frequency.

POCT technology benefits also have been realized in many traditional laboratory settings. Decreased sample volume, small analyzer size and portability, ease of use, and fast TAT have made POCT technology a replacement option for laboratory equipment in many traditional laboratories.

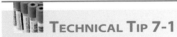

TECHNICAL TIP 7-1

Tests are continually being developed. For an up-to-date listing of POCTs, refer to www.cms.hhs.gov/CLIA/.

PHASES OF LABORATORY TESTING

Laboratory testing is performed in three phases. These are referred to as preexamination, examination, and postexamination. They were previously referred to as preanalytic, analytic, and postanalytic. Procedures should be available to the testing operators that address all three phases of testing for each test. The preexamination phase encompasses the test ordering process; patient identification; patient preparation; sample collection,

handling, and preparation; reagent storage; preparing materials, equipment, and the testing area; and sample application. In the examination phase, the actual test is performed, which includes using correct test codes, test timing, and adding reagents in order. QC is also part of this phase. The final postexamination phase involves interpretation of the test results, recording and reporting results, addressing **critical values** when indicated, following through for confirmatory testing, documenting charges, and biohazard waste disposal. All three phases are vitally important to quality patient testing.

It is important to note that the majority of all laboratory-testing errors in the traditional laboratory occur in the preexamination and postexamination phases of testing; however, POCT errors occur more frequently in the examination phase of testing. Because the technology for most POCT is designed to be user friendly, the potential of performing a test incorrectly and the direct impact of that error are often underestimated. POCT traditionally provides a very short TAT from the collection of the sample to the time a result is obtained. Throughout the very brief testing process, care must be taken throughout all three phases of testing to ensure a timely, quality test result every time. Failure to address just one of several critical steps in each testing process can lead to a negative patient outcome brought about by reporting a fast, but incorrect, result.

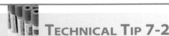

TECHNICAL TIP 7-2

Patient identification must be verified at the bedside and entered correctly in the point-of-care testing device.

Preexamination Phase

Patient identification is the primary concern prior to performing any laboratory test. Because of the nature of POCT, many times no collection tube or sample cup is required to contain the sample prior to performing the test. Although this is perceived as an advantage and can decrease the time it takes to perform a test, it also eliminates one of the traditional audit trails used to verify positive patient identification. Many new POCT devices enable the operator to enter the patient identification into the POCT device, so that the information is captured and stored electronically. Newer technology also has the ability to capture patient identification and operator identification using a bar-code scanner. Failure to identify the patient correctly in the POCT device can result in failure to document a test result that was used to treat or not treat a patient, or the results may be reported on the wrong patient. Both of these scenarios could result in a negative outcome for the patient.

Other preexamination variables that can affect patient outcomes include correct sample collection and proper storage of equipment and supplies. Many POCT supplies have very specific storage requirements. Many are sensitive to heat, light, and moisture. Others require refrigeration and warm-up to room temperature prior to use. The expiration date for some testing supplies changes when they are moved from refrigerated storage to room temperature, or whenever the primary container is opened. No testing supplies should be used past their expiration dates.

TECHNICAL TIP 7-3

Careful attention to collection technique and sample application to the test device is critical for point-of-care coagulation tests.

Examination Phase

The examination phase is the phase at which the actual test is performed. For all POCT, it is imperative that manufacturers' instructions are followed. Application of the sample to the test device and test timing are common errors associated with the examination phase. For some tests, especially coagulation methods, the time between the actual collection of the sample and application to the POCT device is critical, because coagulation starts immediately after the blood sample is removed from the patient.

Test methods that employ a color formation are especially sensitive to critical timing. A test that is read too early or too late can be misinterpreted owing to the lack of color development, color overdevelopment, or degradation of the color that is to be measured. Although POCT devices are designed to be portable, many cannot be moved when analyzing a sample, because movement may disrupt the flow of sample through the device.

Many POCT devices, both automated and manual test kit methods, have built-in procedural QC mechanisms to monitor the examination phase of testing and

alert the operator that a test is invalid or the device simply does not display a test result. Kit methods often include a "control" line that indicates whether the test has been performed correctly. If the control line does not appear, the test is invalid and the patient result cannot be interpreted or reported. The invalid test may be caused by compromised integrity of the testing supplies or addition of test reagents in the wrong order.

TECHNICAL TIP 7-4

Incorrect patient results may be obtained if the test procedure is not followed exactly according to the test package insert and device owner's manual.

Postexamination Phase

The postexamination phase of testing is the interpretation and documentation of the results.

POCT results can be qualitative, semiquantitative, or quantitative. Qualitative results are reported as positive or negative and indicate whether a substance is present or not in the sample. A urine pregnancy test is an example of a qualitative test, because the result is reported as either positive or negative. Semiquantitative results are reported in terms of reaction intensity (1+, 2+, 3+) that equates to a range of numeric values. Quantitative results are numeric results, such as a whole blood glucose result of 99 mg/dL.

TECHNICAL TIP 7-5

Follow manufacturers' storage requirements for reagent strips. Most testing strips may not be stored in an open container and exposed to light, moisture, or heat.

Many POCT devices have the capability to capture results electronically and transmit those results to the permanent medical record. Not all health-care facilities, however, are able to fully use these features.

Manual documentation of POCT results is common. When manual documentation is employed, duplicate transcription is often required to document the result in the patient's permanent medical record and on a laboratory log. The patient's full name, unique identifier, date and time of result, testing operator, location, and test results are required documentation. Results are customarily reported with normal patient **reference ranges,** although it also is common to include therapeutic ranges for most coagulation results **(Fig. 7-1).** A written record of lot numbers and expiration dates for supplies also may be required, depending on the test complexity and accrediting organization **(Fig. 7-2).**

In some cases, even after the documentation is completed, the testing process is not finished. POCT staff also must be familiar with the critical values for each test and the processes for notification of attending staff and/or initiating treatment adjustments. For some POCTs, a result may require confirmatory testing. The confirmatory testing process may include obtaining an additional order, patient consent, and/or collection of a new sample. Finally, the operator must properly dispose of all biohazard items.

TECHNICAL TIP 7-6

When working for a different organization, do not assume that you will be using the same procedure kits. Read the package inserts for all kits and instruments before performing tests.

TECHNICAL TIP 7-7

The Joint Commission mandates that point-of-care tests be classified as a screening or definitive test.

QUALITY CONTROL

The purpose of QC is to ensure the accuracy, precision, and reliability of the test system. Specific QC information regarding the type of control sample, preparation and handling, frequency of use, tolerance levels, and method of recording the QC results are included in the procedure for each test. QC procedures verify the functional integrity of the testing supplies and the POCT device. QC also confirms that the testing operator can perform the test correctly. Additionally, QC testing must

be performed to satisfy regulatory requirements. Regulations governing all laboratory testing require that patient test results must correlate with QC results. This means that a laboratory must be able to prove that the reliability of the test system was confirmed each day that a patient test was performed. Successful QC performance ensures that the operator can use the test system to perform patient testing and that the patient result will be valid. If the QC results are within the specified performance range, meaning the QC results are the expected answers, then the operator also can test a patient sample and get a quality result. The operator has controlled the quality of the test system.

Light, moisture, cleaning agents, or premature deterioration can affect POCT supplies. QC testing verifies the integrity of the testing device and testing supplies and confirms that the test is performing properly for each patient test. QC testing also may be indicated after POCT device maintenance, any time a POCT device has been dropped, or if patient results do not match the patient symptoms.

External Controls

External QCs are tested in the same manner as a patient sample and are used to verify test systems that use urine or blood samples. The external commercial controls are manufactured samples with known values, and they are available in several strengths, such as abnormal low, normal, and abnormal high ranges or positive and negative depending on the test being performed. At least two levels of assayed control are used daily to evaluate performance of instruments. External controls for POCT methods are required each time a new test kit is opened, or with each new lot and each new shipment of testing supplies.

In January 2014, the Centers for Medicare & Medicaid Services (CMS) in accordance with the Clinical and Laboratory Standards Institute (CLSI) guideline EP-23 offers a second option for QC called an Individualized Quality Control Plan (IQCP) that includes a risk assessment (RA), a quality control plan (QCP), and a quality assessment (QA). With this option, the laboratory will determine the frequency of QC based on information about the test, the risk assessment, and accreditation agencies' requirements.

Internal Controls

Internal controls are part of or built into the test system and may be called procedural controls. Internal controls

LABORATORY REPORT FORM

Patient Name: _____   Test Date: _____

Patient ID: _____

Test	Results	Reference Ranges
Urinalysis (adult)	Clean Catch YES NO	
Specific gravity		1.001–1.030
pH		5–6
Leukocytes		Neg
Nitrate		Neg
Protein (mg/dL)	mg/dL	Neg
Glucose (mg/dL)	mg/dL	Neg
Ketone		Neg
Urobilinogen (mg/dL)	mg/dL	<1
Bilirubin		Neg
Blood (RBC/uL)	RBC/uL	Neg
Stool for Occult Blood	Internal Pos/Neg Controls: OK	Neg
Hemoglobin by HemoCue (g/dL)	g/dL	4 to 10 months 10.0–14.0 g/dL
		10 mo to 3 yrs 11.0–14.0 g/dL
		4 to 9 yrs 11.5–15.0 g/dL
		9 to 14 yrs 12.0–15.6 g/dL
		Adult Female 11.6–16.1 g/dL
		Adult Male 13.3–17.7 g/dL
Mono Test	Internal Pos/Neg Controls: OK	Neg
Rapid Strep A/Throat	Internal Pos/Neg Controls: OK	Neg
Glucose (Whole Blood)	mg/dL	70–99 mg/dL (fasting)
		If patient not fasting—
		Time of last food intake:
		Time of test: _____
Urine Pregnancy Test (hCG)	Internal Pos/Neg Controls: OK	Neg (LMP)
Vaginal Wet Prep/KOH		Neg
(PPMP, performed only by		
Nurse Practitioner)		
Comments:		

Person performing test (Initial): _____   Practitioner: _____

FIGURE 7-1 Laboratory report form with reference ranges.

SURESTEP WHOLE BLOOD GLUCOSE
PATIENT/QUALITY CONTROL LOG

Test Strip Lot # _____   Control Code: _____   Exp. Date: _____
Low Control Lot # _____ Low Control QC Range: _____   Exp. Date: _____
High Control Lot # _____ High Control QC Range: _____   Exp. Date: _____

DATE	PATIENT NAME (Or use patient label)	PATIENT ID	PATIENT RESULT	LOW CONTROL	HIGH CONTROL	TECH

Reviewed by: _____   Date: _____

FIGURE 7-2 SureStep whole blood glucose patient/QC log.

are commonly used in test kit systems to verify that the test kit and any added reagents performed as expected. Many waived tests have internal procedure controls that indicate that the test was performed correctly and that it was completed. Internal controls are performed with each test.

Electronic Controls

Electronic controls monitor the test system's electronic components. This type of control can be internal or external, depending on the device.

Many test systems use a combination of external and internal controls to verify the entire test system is working properly. Some POCT devices have a safety feature that locks the meter to prevent any patient testing until the QC error is resolved.

Documentation of QC

Documentation of QC testing is required. Some POCT devices can capture this information electronically, and other methods require manual documentation. When interpreting the QC result, it is imperative to verify that the controls performed as expected. Any time a QC result does not perform as expected (the results are not within the predetermined range), no further patient testing should be performed until the QC error is corrected. The test procedure should provide guidance to resolve the error. Additional guidance can be obtained from the test manufacturer. Documentation of successful QC performance is required to confirm that the test system was able to produce valid test results on the same day that patient testing was performed **(Fig. 7-3).**

TECHNICAL TIP 7-8

Patient test results can never be reported if the QC test results are not in the specified range. The problem must be resolved and the test repeated.

PROCEDURES

The CLIA requires that operators performing POCT follow manufacturers' guidelines and that written test procedures must be available to all testing personnel. It is important to understand that POCT procedures vary among manufacturers; therefore, package inserts and procedures in the procedure manual are not interchangeable. The procedure manual must be updated when a facility changes to a different manufacturer. Testing personnel must read the entire package insert or procedure manual before performing the test.

TECHNICAL TIP 7-9

Written test procedures must be available to all testing personnel.

The information in package inserts includes the purpose of the test, identifies who may perform the test, sample collection, handling, and preservation, safety precautions, instrument maintenance and **calibration,** reagent storage requirements, QC requirements, procedural steps, interpretation of results and reference values, and sources of error. Manufacturers also provide training materials and assistance in troubleshooting technical problems.

Areas in which POCT is performed are required to maintain a procedure manual that is readily available to all testing personnel. The procedure manual contains the information provided in the package inserts from the instrumentation, reagents, and controls for each procedure, the purpose of the test, and identifies who may perform the test. It also contains site-specific information, such as the location of supplies, special handling requirements, patient identification procedures for devices with connectivity, instructions for reporting and recording results, and the protocol to follow when critically low or high test results are encountered.

TECHNICAL TIP 7-10

Recorded results must be legible, in a location where they may be reviewed by the health-care provider, and easily retrieved when needed.

All patient test results must be recorded in the patient's permanent medical record. The patient test result must include the patient name and identification number, the initials of the operator who performed the

URINE DIPSTICK QUALITY CONTROL LOG
for
Chemstrip 10

Quality Control **Level 2 (Abnormal) Lot #** __44461__   Quality Control Exp. Date __01/14/16__

Reagent lot # _____   Reagent Exp. Date _____

Date	Sp. Gravity	pH	Leuko	Nitrite	Protein	Glucose	Ketones	Urobil	Bilirubin	Blood	Tech
QC Range	1.000−1.015	7−9	Tr−2+	Pos	30−500 (1+−3+)	100−1000	1+−3+	Pos	1+−3+	Tr−250 (tr−3+)	

POCT-5   Reviewed _____

FIGURE 7-3 Example of urine dipstick QC log for Chemstrip 10 (abnormal control).

test, the date the test was performed, and the facility where the test was performed. In many cases, the hospital computer system will capture this information when patient test results are entered.

COMMON POCT ERRORS

One statistic of interest is that laboratory test results influence approximately 70 percent of medical decisions. A common misconception is that POCT can be performed with minimal or no training because many POCTs are only screening tests and the techniques to perform a test are usually quite simple. It is important to understand that whether tests are only for screening or are used to monitor ongoing therapy, they have value. If the test were of no value, it would not be needed. Each result has the potential to shape a patient's outcome in a positive or negative way, and incorrect results can negatively affect patient care, treatment, and outcome. The following scenario illustrates examples of possible negative outcomes for a qualitative urine dipstick test to identify blood in urine.

Preexamination failure: Failure to obtain the sample from the correct patient and/or failure to label the sample with the correct patient name would mean that the right results would be charted on the wrong patient. Failure to collect the sample in a clean container may cause a false-positive test because bleach residue can cause a false-positive result for blood.

Examination failure: Failure to perform QC could cause a wrong result if the test strips had been compromised because the test strip integrity was not verified. Failure to read the test strip at the correct time by interpreting the result too early could result in the difference between a negative or positive screening result.

Postexamination failure: Failure to document the result in the medical record may result in questioning the medical necessity of a confirmatory test. A result that drives a treatment plan must be recorded in the permanent medical record.

All incorrect results can affect the patient outcome by influencing the way the patient is treated, or not treated, and the sequence of ordering additional diagnostic tests based on that simple screening test. **Table 7-2** lists the common errors associated with POCT.

TABLE 7-2 Common Errors Associated with POCT

Tests	Errors
Hemoglobin	Failure to adequately fill the cuvette Bubbles in the cuvette
Glucose	Use of compromised or expired reagent strips Failure to adequately cleanse and dry the capillary puncture site Failure to adequately or correctly apply sample to testing area Failure to run controls and document results as required
iSTAT profiles	Failure to identify the patient correctly in the meter Failure to observe cartridge warm-up time Failure to comply with room-temperature expiration dates Returning room-temperature cartridges to refrigerated storage Underfilled or overfilled cartridges Squeezing the cartridge when closing Moving the device while analyzing a sample Failure to upload meter for timely data transfer
Urinalysis	Leaving the urine sample at room temperature for more than 2 hours without a preservative Use of compromised or expired reagent strips Incorrect reaction timing Leaving reagent strips in the sample too long Exposing test strips to heat, light, moisture, and cleaning agents
Occult blood (guaiac slide methods)	Failure to use the correct sample type for the test kit Failure to apply the correct amount of sample on the slide Failure to wait specified time after sample is applied to add the developer reagent Patients not given precollection instructions

TABLE 7-2 Common Errors Associated with POCT—cont'd

Tests	Errors
Toxicology profile	Use of incorrectly stored or expired kits Misinterpretation of patient and control results
Group A *Streptococcus*	Use of cotton or calcium alginate collection swabs Use of compromised or expired reagent kits Failure to observe the internal control Incorrect collection or timing
Urine pregnancy test	Failure to test a first morning sample Addition of reagents in the wrong order Misinterpretation of test and control results
Immunoassay kits	Using reagents from different kits Failure to follow the step-by-step instructions Use of incorrectly stored or expired kits Misinterpretation of test and control results Failure to observe and document internal control results
POC meters (analyzers) with data management	Failure to identify the patient correctly in the meter Failure to follow correct timing for application of sample to test strip/test cartridge Failure to follow correct timing for placing test strip/test cartridge in the meter Failure to upload meter for timely data transfer
Coagulation tests	Failure to adequately cleanse and dry the capillary puncture site Failure to follow manufacturer's instructions for sample collection Failure to match code chip and code number on test strip vial Prematurely performing the capillary puncture before test strip/test cartridge is ready to accept the sample Inadequate application of sample

TECHNICAL TIP 7-11

The test result is only as good as the sample collected!!

TECHNICAL TIP 7-12

Anytime a result does not match a patient's clinical symptoms, or there are other indications that the result may not be valid, repeat the test.

Critical Elements: The Magnificent Seven

Each time a POCT is performed; there are multiple opportunities to make an error that could result in a negative patient outcome. It is impossible to list all of the sources of error and the resulting outcome for the ever-growing list of POCTs. **Box 7-1** lists the critical elements for good laboratory practice that, when followed, will prevent the majority of common POCT errors.

SAFETY

As health-care professionals, patient safety and the safety of the POCT operator are the responsibility of the POCT operator. Standard precautions must be followed for each test procedure. Because POCT may be performed directly at the patient's bedside, care also must be taken to identify and reduce the risk for a POCT device to spread infection between patients. Use of gloves, personal protective equipment, hand sanitizing, and POCT device cleaning maintenance protocol must be strictly followed. Additionally, care must be taken to protect patients, staff, and POCT devices in both protective and infection isolation environments.

BOX 7-1 Critical Elements: The Magnificent Seven

1. Patient identification—Identify the correct patient. Use the full name and a second identifier on all samples, requisitions, and reports.
2. Proper sample collection—Ensure the correct sample type is collected, use correct collection technique, label all samples, and handle and transport samples according to procedure.
3. Proper storage of testing supplies—Store reagents at the correct storage temperature and never use an expired test reagent or collection device.
4. QC—Always perform and document QC as required and confirm that QC results are within the expected range before any patient testing is performed.
5. Sample application and test performance— Always follow manufacturers' instructions for applying the sample to the test device and strictly follow test-timing instructions.
6. Result interpretation—Refer to the test procedure for correct interpretation of test result, confirmatory testing that may be required, and guidance for identification and communication of critical results.
7. Documentation of results—Results must be recorded in the permanent medical record, legible, and easily retrieved.

QUALITY MANAGEMENT AND REGULATORY COMPLIANCE

Quality management is a comprehensive, multifaceted process used to monitor, evaluate, and improve the quality of laboratory services through all three phases of patient testing. The purpose of quality management is to achieve the highest level of excellence in patient care. It is made of many elements.

All laboratory testing is regulated by the federal law, the Clinical Laboratory Improvement Act (CLIA), and is enforced by the CMS. CLIA defines the standards and guidelines for performing POCT and all other laboratory testing. Accrediting organizations, such as the College of American Pathologists (CAP), The Joint Commission (TJC), the Commission on Laboratory Accreditation (COLA), the American Association of Blood Banks (AABB), and the Food and Drug Administration (FDA) must follow the minimum requirements for laboratory practice required by CLIA. Accrediting organization standards customarily have more stringent regulatory requirements than CLIA. It is important to understand that the regulations, however ominous they may seem, are in place to provide a minimum standard of quality for all laboratory testing. Compliance with CLIA and accrediting organizations' regulatory standards is mandatory and is normally evaluated using a biannual inspection process. Failure to comply with the regulatory standards can lead to federal sanctions, and loss of accreditation and the ability to legally perform all laboratory testing.

Laboratory testing is classified into four complexity categories: waived, moderate complexity, high complexity, and provider-performed microscopy procedures (PPMP). Most POCT is waived, moderate complexity, or PPMP. The complexity is assigned by the FDA and is based on the skill level required to perform the test. Test complexity is determined by the testing characteristics such as stability of the reagent, preparation of the reagent, operational steps, calibration, and QC. Complexity also depends on the degree of knowledge, training, experience, troubleshooting, and interpretation required in the testing process. The complexity test performed determines the level of certification required.

Waived Tests

Waived tests are defined as procedures that employ methodologies that are easy to perform, and the likelihood of erroneous results is negligible. Waived tests are considered simple to perform and interpret, require no special training or education background, and require only minimum QC. To perform waived testing, the organization must obtain a Certificate of Waiver from the CMS and follow manufacturers' directions for the testing process. Many waived tests, such as glucose monitoring and pregnancy tests, are available over the counter to all consumers.

Moderate Complexity

Moderate-complexity tests are more difficult to perform than are waived tests and require documentation of training in testing principles, instrument calibration, and QC. Moderate-complexity testing requires that testing personnel have a minimum of a high school diploma or equivalent. Facilities performing moderate-complexity tests are subject to proficiency testing and on-site inspections.

High Complexity

High-complexity tests require sophisticated instrumentation and a high degree of interpretation by testing personnel. High-complexity testing requires operators with specific laboratory science education, or they can be performed by staff who meet the moderate-complexity requirements provided the testing is directly supervised by a laboratory professional.

Provider-Performed Microscopy Procedures

This category includes clinical microscopy procedures. Facilities performing these tests must meet the moderate-complexity requirements for proficiency testing, patient test management, and QC as required by the accreditation agency. PPMP tests may be performed only by licensed providers, such as physicians, nurse practitioners, physician assistants, midwives, and dentists during a patient's examination.

Training and Competency Assessment

All POCT operators must receive training prior to performing patient testing. Competency assessment ensures testing procedures are performed consistently and accurately. Training and competency assessment must encompass the three phases of testing. Competency can be evaluated by methods such as observation, evaluating adequacy of documentation, or blind test of samples with known values, such as QC materials, **proficiency testing** samples, or previously analyzed patient samples, and written quizzes.

Competency assessment is required by CLIA regulations for all POCT operators who perform moderate- and high-complexity testing at 6 months and 1 year after initial training. After the first year, competency must be assessed and validated annually. Most accrediting agencies also require annual competency assessment for staff performing waived tests.

TECHNICAL TIP 7-13

Failure to comply with mandatory regulatory standards can lead to federal sanctions and/or loss of accreditation.

POCT FUTURE

The future of POCT will be driven by the increased demand for rapid testing and a broader scope of clinically relevant information. POC device technology will continue to develop portable, stand-alone devices with diverse test menus. Robust data management and connectivity to the patient electronic medical record will become the standard of care. New therapies also will force the evolution of new tests and test methods including noninvasive and alternative sample technologies. Health care, in general, is a dynamic profession and change in this field is constant. POCT will continue to play an increasing role in providing quality results in diverse patient care environments.

BIBLIOGRAPHY

CLSI: *Laboratory Quality Control Based on Risk Management; Approved Guideline.* CLSI document EP23A. Wayne, PA, CLSI, 2011.

Njoroge, S., and Nichols, J.: Managing risk at the point-of-care: Preventing errors. *Clinical Laboratory News*, July 2014.

Strasinger, S.K., and Di Lorenzo, M.S.: *The Phlebotomy Textbook*, ed. 3. Philadelphia, F.A. Davis, 2011.

INTERNET RESOURCES

www.phppo.cdc.gov/clia/default.asp

www.fda.gov/cdrh/CLIA/index.html

www.cms.hhs.gov/CLIA/

wwwn.cdc.gov/dls/bestpractices/

www.cdc.gov/clia/

www.accessdata.fda.gov/scripts/cdrh/cfdocs/cfCLIA/search.cfm

www.osha.gov/SLTC/etools/hospital/lab/lab.html#OSHA_Laboratory_Standard

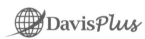 For additional material, please visit **http://davisplus.fadavis.com.**

REVIEW QUESTIONS

1. **Which of the following are preexamination errors in POCT?**
   a. Improper storage of test materials
   b. Failure to check reagent expiration dates
   c. Performing the test on the wrong patient
   d. All of the above

2. **QC is part of the:**
   a. Preexamination phase
   b. Examination phase
   c. Postexamination phase
   d. Collection phase

3. **Test result documentation is part of the:**
   a. Preexamination phase
   b. Examination phase
   c. Laboratory phase
   d. Postexamination phase

4. **Procedural controls that verify that the test kit and added reagents are performing correctly are called:**
   a. Electronic controls
   b. External controls
   c. Internal controls
   d. Proficiency testing

5. **Acceptable QC can ensure:**
   a. Correct functioning of the testing device
   b. Integrity of the testing materials
   c. Correct performance of the test
   d. All of the above

6. **The two levels of control samples that are tested to ensure test result accuracy are:**
   a. Baseline and elevated
   b. Normal and abnormal
   c. Acceptable and unacceptable
   d. Internal and proficiency

7. **To determine the proper maintenance of a POCT instrument, the operator should:**
   a. Attend a proficiency class
   b. Read the package insert
   c. Contact the manufacturer
   d. Consult with another caregiver

8. **When performing POCT, the operator must be sure to document results of:**
   a. Patient tests
   b. Quality control
   c. Reference ranges
   d. All of the above

9. **Errors most commonly associated with incorrect PT/INR results are:**
   a. Failure to adequately cleanse and dry the capillary puncture site
   b. Prematurely performing the capillary puncture before the test strip/cartridge is ready to accept the sample
   c. Inadequate application of sample
   d. All of the above

10. Six months after beginning employment, a health-care worker is given a sample by the POCT supervisor and asked to perform a screening test for group A *Streptococcus* and return the results to the supervisor. The employee is performing:
    a. QC
    b. Compliance testing
    c. Patient testing
    d. Competency testing

FOR FURTHER STUDY

1. Define QC and explain why it is required before any patient testing.

2. Explain what has happened when a POCT instrument goes into a locking mode and does not allow the operator to continue with the procedure.

3. Indicate whether each of the following actions is acceptable or not acceptable POCT technique and explain why an action is unacceptable.
    a. A POCT operator is performing a microscopic analysis of urine in an office with a Certificate of Waiver for waived testing complexity.
    b. The POCT operator records the lot number and expiration date of a control on the QC log sheet.
    c. When performing a test for occult blood using the guaiac slide method, the operator immediately applies the developer reagent to the slide after applying the fecal sample.
    d. The POCT operator performs a QuickVue In-Line Strep A test using a cartridge from one test kit and extraction solution from a different manufacturer's kit.

CASE STUDY 7-1

Anne, the nurse, performed the daily morning QC on the glucose meter. The results were:
Abnormal low = 50 mg/dL
Abnormal high = 200 mg/dL

The range for the abnormal low is 33 to 57 mg/dL; the abnormal high range is 278 to 418 mg/dL.

1. Can Anne report patient results?
2. What actions are required by Anne?
3. What is a possible cause of any discrepancy?

CASE STUDY 7-2

Laurie, a medical assistant, received a urine sample from the patient at 0900 and placed it on the counter in the physician's office laboratory. Because of the number of patients with whom Anne was working that morning, she did not get back to the laboratory to perform the urinalysis on this sample until 1300. The results were:

Color: Yellow	Protein: Negative	Bilirubin: Negative
Clarity: Cloudy*	Glucose: Negative	Urobilinogen: Normal
Sp. Gravity: 1.020	Ketones: Negative	Nitrite: Positive*
pH: 9.0*	Blood: Negative	Leukocyte: Negative

*Significant results

1. What could be a possible cause for the abnormal results?
2. What should have been done with this sample?
3. What will Anne have to do?

EVALUATION OF A POINT-OF-CARE TEST

RATING SYSTEM

2 = Satisfactory

1 = Needs improvement

0 = Incorrect/did not perform

_____ 1. Removes the test kit from the refrigerator and allows the reagents to warm to room temperature, if required.

_____ 2. Checks the expiration date of the kit.

_____ 3. Turns the instrument on for the correct amount of warm-up time according to manufacturer's instructions.

_____ 4. Performs QC according to facility protocol and manufacturer's instructions.

_____ 5. Identifies the patient using two identifiers, explains the procedure, and obtains consent.

_____ 6. Sanitizes hands and puts on gloves.

_____ 7. Obtains the sample according to manufacturer's instructions.

_____ 8. Performs the test following the manufacturer's directions.

_____ 9. Interprets the test results according to the provided interpretation chart.

_____ 10. Records results and reference ranges according to facility protocol.

_____ 11. Cleanses work area and instrument following OSHA guidelines.

_____ 12. Follows instrument directions for additional testing and/or turning off instrument.

_____ 13. Performs any post-sample collection procedures on the patient.

_____ 14. Removes the gloves and sanitizes hands .

_____ 15. Thanks the patient.

TOTAL POINTS

MAXIMUM POINTS = 30

COMMENTS:

Blood Collection From Vascular Access Devices

LEARNING OBJECTIVES

Upon completion of this chapter, the reader will be able to:

8.1 Discuss the correct selection and use of equipment necessary for insertion and maintenance of peripheral access devices.

8.2 Explain the preparation of the venous access site, insertion of the catheter, and connection of the IV fluids to the catheter.

8.3 Describe the blood collection procedure from peripheral vascular access devices.

8.4 List the various types of central venous catheters (CVCs) and describe the purpose of each.

8.5 Describe the blood collection procedures using CVCs following laboratory protocol and the correct order of draw.

INTRODUCTION

Advances in the delivery of medications have produced an increase in patients receiving direct venous infusion of medications. These changes have resulted in the need to use additional methods for the collection of blood samples.

This chapter describes the **peripheral access devices** and the various **central venous catheters** (CVCs) and the correct method for collecting blood from each. Different procedures are required for the various devices and knowledge of each is necessary to collect a quality blood sample while maintaining the integrity of the device.

PERIPHERAL ACCESS DEVICES

Introduction

Peripheral access devices, including peripheral IV lines and midline peripheral catheters, are commonly used in hospitals and clinics to administer medications and IV fluids directly into the circulatory system.

The peripheral IV insertion procedure is performed under aseptic technique, using a selected IV catheter that is inserted through the skin into a vein. IV catheters come in a variety of sizes ranging from 14 gauge to 24 gauge: the smaller the gauge number, the larger the catheter size. It is recommended to choose the smallest size and shortest length to accommodate the prescribed therapy. In an emergency situation, a larger catheter size may be used, such as a 16 or 18 gauge. The most common, all-purpose IV catheter size is a 20 gauge. It is essential for health-care providers to understand the techniques and be proficient in obtaining and maintaining IV access for continuum of care of their patients.

The midline peripheral catheter is defined as a catheter that is between 3 inches and 8 inches in length.

It is inserted above or below the antecubital fossa, with the tip terminating distal to the shoulder. These catheters are inserted by specially trained health-care professionals. Midline catheters are designed for intermediate-term therapies of 2 or more weeks.

 TECHNICAL TIP 8-1

Unlike the procedures for blood collection from CVCs, blood for laboratory testing is drawn only from peripheral access devices at the time of their insertion.

 SAFETY TIP 8-1

Follow strict hand-washing guidelines and maintain sterile technique throughout the process.

 TECHNICAL TIP 8-2

When pulling back on the syringe, confirm that the blood flows back easily and that it is easy to flush back into the vein.

 SAFETY TIP 8-2

It is very important to secure IV tubing to the patient and to explain precautions related to unassisted ambulation to the patient.

BLOOD COLLECTION FROM PERIPHERAL VASCULAR ACCESS DEVICES (PERIPHERAL IVs)

Blood sample collection from a peripheral vascular access device is performed only at the time of initial insertion of the device. Do not collect blood samples from indwelling peripheral or midline catheters. At the time

PROCEDURE 8-1 Peripheral IV Insertion

EQUIPMENT:

Gloves
Tourniquet (single use/latex-free)
Chlorhexidine gluconate sponge
Iodine and alcohol pads (optional)
IV catheter device
IV tubing and solution

One 10-mL saline flush syringe
One-way valve connector device
Occlusive dressing
Tape—two to three ¼-inch strips
2 × 2 gauze pads

PROCEDURE:

Step 1. Introduce yourself and explain the procedure. Allow the patient the opportunity to ask questions and to verbalize understanding.

Step 2. Identify the patient verbally by having him or her state both the first name and last name, and date of birth. Compare the information on the patient's ID band with the requisition form.

Step 3. Sanitize your hands, put on gloves, and prepare the equipment needed for insertion.

Step 4. Choose the appropriate size catheter.

Step 5. Collect the necessary supplies and equipment. It may be helpful to place a disposable pad down first on the work surface, to help keep equipment and supplies clean and organized.

Step 6. Verify the type of IV fluid that is to be administered.

Step 7. Fill the drip chamber halfway, prime the tubing to remove any air bubbles, and close the clamp. Examine the IV bag and tubing for leaks.

Step 8. Remove gloves and sanitize hands. Put on new gloves.

Step 9. Connect the saline flush syringe to the one-way valve connector device and flush with 1 mL of solution. Leave the end cap on the connector device to maintain sterility.

Step 10. To position the patient, hyperextend the patient's arm and place an absorbent pad or towel under the arm to prevent soiling of the bed linen.

Step 11. Apply the tourniquet about 4 to 6 inches above the puncture site. Palpate the vein to determine its location and direction.

Step 12. Scrub site vigorously with a chlorhexidine gluconate sponge for 30 seconds to sterilize the site. Alternately, the site can be wiped with an alcohol pad in a circular motion, followed by an iodine swab. Start in a circular motion, from the puncture site working outward approximately 1½ to 2 inches. Allow the iodine to dry completely (30 to 60 seconds).

Step 13. Remove the catheter from the package and inspect quickly for any defect on the outside of the catheter. Anchor the vein with nondominant hand, and grasp catheter firmly between the thumb and index finger of the dominant hand with bevel of the needle inside the catheter pointed up at a 15- to 30-degree angle.

Step 14. Insert the tip of the catheter into the vein, observing for a flashback of blood into the small chamber of the catheter. Once a flashback is observed, start advancing the catheter using the thumb while holding the catheter in place with the index finger. Some health-care professionals use a two-handed technique, by advancing with one hand, while the other hand holds the catheter in place. The catheter will advance easier when the vein remains anchored and skin traction

PROCEDURE 8-1 Peripheral IV Insertion (Continued)

is maintained. Both methods are considered adequate for successful insertion.

Step 15. When the catheter is inserted into the vein, remove the tourniquet. Remove the needle device (stylet) by gently twisting to unscrew the needle device from the catheter while applying light pressure to the top of the catheter. Connect the one-way connector with the flush syringe or blood collection syringe attached.

Step 16. If laboratory tests are not ordered, flush with 2 to 3 mL of sterile saline solution and pull back to check blood return. Blood collection from a peripheral IV is discussed in the following section.

Step 17. While flushing, observe for any signs of swelling in the area or any pain the patient may be experiencing.

Step 18. Once adequate blood flow and flushing have been established, secure the device

with tape, over and around the catheter. Place a sterile occlusive dressing to cover the entire insertion site.

Step 19. Attach the IV fluids to the device, open clamps, and run fluids as ordered.

Step 20. Label the occlusive dressing with the date, time, catheter size, and initials.

Step 21. Follow facility's policies regarding maintenance.

Step 22. Dispose of all sharps into an approved sharps container. Other materials can be placed into the nonbiohazard waste container.

Step 23. Remove gloves, sanitize hands, and thank the patient.

Step 24. The IV site should be inspected daily for any signs of redness, drainage, and swelling.

of insertion blood may be collected prior to administration of treatment. Refer to step 15 of Procedure 8-1, Peripheral IV Insertion.

Blood can be collected by attaching an appropriate size syringe or syringes to the catheter connector and slowly withdrawing the required amount of blood. The blood is then transferred to the required evacuated tubes using a blood transfer device. Blood from the catheter connector also can be collected directly into evacuated tubes and a tube holder.

 TECHNICAL TIP 8-3

Always use a transfer device when filling tubes from a syringe. Attaching a needle to the syringe and puncturing the evacuated tube stopper not only is dangerous to the collector but also may result in hemolysis of the sample.

CENTRAL VENOUS CATHETERS

Introduction

CVCs are a special type of catheter that is inserted by a physician or a certified health-care professional as either an internal catheter or external catheter into a large vessel of the body. CVCs are used when an individual requires long-term medication administration (antibiotics or chemotherapy) or nutritional support. CVCs also are considered when the patient's vasculature prohibits placing a peripheral IV and frequent blood draws are warranted. The choice of what type and whether it is an internal or external catheter depends on the specific patient need and preference of the health-care professional inserting the catheter.

Types

There are four types of CVCs: (1) nontunneled, noncuffed; (2) tunneled; (3) implanted; and (4) a peripherally inserted central catheter (PICC).

PROCEDURE 8-2 Blood Sample Collection From a Peripheral Venous Access

EQUIPMENT:

Gloves	Injection cap, if needed
One 10-mL syringe	Alcohol wipes
0.9 percent sterile saline	Male/female sterile cap

PROCEDURE:

Step 1. Introduce yourself and explain the procedure, and obtain consent.

Step 2. Identify the patient verbally by having him or her state both the first name and last name, and date of birth. Compare the information on the patient's ID band with the requisition form.

Step 3. Sanitize your hands, put on gloves, and prepare the equipment needed for blood collection.

Step 4. Blood will be collected from the appropriate vein for intended infusion therapy because the catheter will be left in place **(see Procedure 8-1).**

Step 5. When the vein is accessed and catheter is advanced into the vein until the hub rests at the venipuncture site, apply transparent dressing over catheter.

Step 6. Using index and middle finger of nondominant hand, apply pressure over tip of catheter to occlude blood flow.

Step 7. Remove stylet and attach syringe.

Step 8. Withdraw amount of blood requested for laboratory tests.

Step 9. Transfer blood using a blood transfer device into the appropriate tubes following the correct order of draw. Mix tubes by gentle inversion (three to eight times) immediately.

Step 10. Attach loop and flush with 8 to 9 mL of saline. Attach appropriate tubing for IV infusion.

Step 11. If using an evacuated tube system:
a. Attach blunt cannula of tube holder into catheter adapter.
b. Advance sample tube on to stopper-puncturing needle in the holder.
c. Observe for flow of blood into the tube.
d. Allow tube to fill.
e. If more than one tube of blood is needed, change tubes slowly and steadily, taking care not to move catheter in cannulated vein and cause the patient undue pain or discomfort. Fill the tubes in the correct order of draw.
f. Mix tubes immediately for the correct number of inversions as they are removed from the holder.
g. Remove holder and continue with the original procedure (see Procedure 8-1).

Nontunneled, Noncuffed Central Catheter

This type of catheter is inserted directly through the skin and into a large vein in the jugular, subclavian, or femoral veins. It is commonly called a triple-lumen catheter, having one to three ports to access with antireflux valve connector end caps on the ends of ports. After insertion, this catheter is covered with an occlusive waterproof dressing **(see Fig. 8-1).**

Tunneled

A tunneled catheter is surgically placed by a physician by tunneling the catheter under the skin from the vein entry point to an exit site outside on the chest. Broviac, Hickman, and Groshong are examples of tunneled catheters, meaning that part of the catheter is on the outside of the body, with the tip of the catheter placed internally in a large vein just above the heart. These

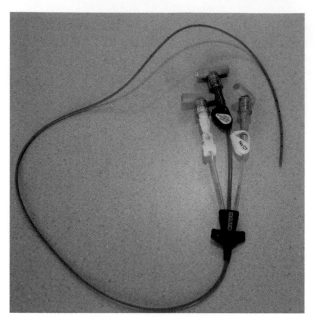

FIGURE 8-1 **Triple-lumen catheter.** *(Reproduced with permission from Strasinger, S.K., and Di Lorenzo, M.S.: The Phlebotomy Textbook, ed. 3. Philadelphia, F.A. Davis, 2011.)*

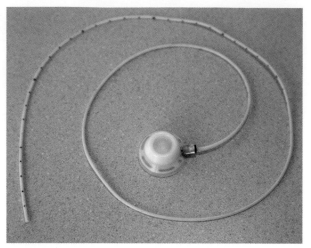

FIGURE 8-2 **Implanted port.** *(Reproduced with permission from Strasinger, S.K., and Di Lorenzo, M.S.: The Phlebotomy Textbook, ed. 3. Philadelphia, F.A. Davis, 2011.)*

require a sterile dressing to be applied over their insertion site.

Hickman catheters may be single- or multilumen. The most common is the double lumen, which has two color-coded tails; the white port is for routine IV fluids and medications and the red port is for blood draws and infusing blood products.

The Groshong catheter is a clear silicone external catheter with a blue radiopaque line running alongside the length of the catheter. This catheter has a three-position valve at the end of the catheter tip. The valve opens to allow blood collection and fluid infusion but does not allow backflow of blood. Therefore, use of heparin is not needed with this type of catheter and is not recommended.

Implanted Port

This implanted device is placed under the skin surgically by a physician. It consists of a self-sealing septum housed in a metal or plastic case, with a catheter that is threaded into the superior vena cava (SVC). The port is palpated to locate the septum, and is accessed with a specially designed **noncoring needle,** often called a Huber needle. This needle has a deflected tip and is configured at a 90-degree angle. This type of port may be a single- or double-lumen catheter. It is commonly used in long-term drug therapies, such as the administration of chemotherapy but also can be used for blood draws **(see Fig. 8-2).**

Peripherally Inserted Central Catheters (PICC Lines)

This type of catheter is inserted through a large peripheral vein of the upper arm into the lower one-third of the superior vena cava (SVC) to the junction of the SVC in the right atrium (SVC/RA). Specially trained health-care professionals insert the catheter by threading the catheter through an introducer needle. There is an injection cap attached to the lumen(s) of the catheter, where the IV is connected or blood samples are removed. This catheter can be left in for several weeks to months.

To obtain blood from a PICC, the catheter size must be 4 French (Fr) or greater in size. If a PICC is being used for total parental nutrition (TPN), it cannot be used for blood drawing. It also is important not to apply a tourniquet or a blood pressure cuff to the arm with the PICC line, because this may occlude or collapse the catheter.

 SAFETY TIP 8-3

PICC line catheters require frequent observations. Assessing insertion site and changing of dressing and injection cap are necessary to avoid infection. Follow your facility's policy regarding manipulation or use of PICC lines.

Flushing peripheral IVs and CVCs is performed to ensure and maintain patency of the catheter and to prevent mixing of medications and solutions that are incompatible. Follow manufacturers' instructions for correct use and institutional policy and procedure for flushing.

Blood Sample Collection

Blood sample collection for laboratory testing, donor collection, or therapeutic indications can be routinely drawn from certain central vascular access devices. However, this procedure must be performed by specially trained personnel. Specific procedures must be followed for flushing the catheters with saline, and possibly heparin, when blood collection is completed. Sterile technique procedures must be strictly adhered to when entering CVCs, because they provide a direct path for infectious organisms to enter the patient's bloodstream.

Blood samples may not be drawn from an infusion administration set or proximal to an existing infusion site. It is necessary that the blood collector is knowledgeable about blood collection and the correct order of draw. Refer to the laboratory for confirmation of order of draw and appropriate collection equipment.

Drawing samples for coagulation tests from a CVC is not recommended; however, if this is necessary, they should be collected after 20 mL of blood has been discarded or used for other tests. The order of tube fill may vary slightly to accommodate the amount of blood that must be drawn before a coagulation test. As with other procedures, blood cultures are always collected first. Blood cultures are drawn from CVCs primarily to detect infection of the catheter tip and should be compared with results drawn from a peripheral vein. If these are ordered, the draw will satisfy the additional discard needed for coagulation tests. Therefore, the order of fill is as follows:

1. First syringe—5 mL, discard
2. Second syringe—blood cultures
3. Third syringe—anticoagulated tubes (light blue, lavender, green, and gray)
4. Clotted tubes (red and serum separator tube)

If blood cultures are not ordered, the coagulation tests (light blue stopper tube) can be collected with a new syringe after the other samples have been collected.

PROCEDURE 8-3 Blood Sample Collection From a Central Venous Access Device

EQUIPMENT:

Requisition form
Gloves
Alcohol wipes or chlorhexidine gluconate sponge
Iodine wipes (optional)
Two 10-mL syringes filled with normal saline, for flush
Two 5-mL syringes
Blood collection tubes for ordered tests
Evacuated tube holder
Syringes for blood collection

Blood transfer device
One or two 5-mL syringe(s) filled with heparinized saline, for flushing after using the saline flush. (Optional)

Refer to your facility's policy regarding the use of heparin flush solutions in central lines.

PROCEDURE:

Step 1. Obtain and review health-care provider's order.

Step 2. Identify the patient verbally by having him or her state both the first name and last

PROCEDURE 8-3   Blood Sample Collection From a Central Venous Access Device (Continued)

name, and date of birth. Compare the information on the patient's ID band with the requisition form.

Step 3. Explain the procedure and obtain the patient's consent.

Step 4. Position the patient in a supine position.

Step 5. Assemble supplies and place within easy reach of the patient.

Step 6. Sanitize hands.

Step 7. Put on gloves.

Step 8. Stop infusions in all lumens for 1 minute prior to drawing sample. If the lumen to be used for laboratory draws has an infusion, cap the tubing with a male/female cap when disconnecting.

Step 9. If using a multilumen catheter, clamp all lumens and withdraw from the proximal lumen of the catheter.

Step 10. Cleanse injection cap with alcohol wipe. Using vigorous friction, scrub on the top and in the grooves for 15 seconds. If the laboratory draw is for a blood culture, scrub the infection cap with an alcohol wipe for 30 seconds.

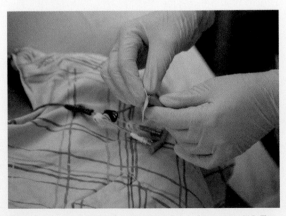

(Reproduced with permission from Strasinger, S.K., and Di Lorenzo, M.S.: The Phlebotomy Textbook, ed. 3. Philadelphia, F.A. Davis, 2011.)

Step 11. Flush with 10 mL of normal saline (if TPN or heparin was infusing, flush line with 20 mL of normal saline).

Step 12. Using the same syringe, withdraw 5 mL of blood. Remove syringe and discard syringe in biohazard container. Wait 10 to 15 seconds to draw the sample.

Step 13. Use a sterile syringe to collect the sample. **Collect the smallest volume amount of blood required for each test.**

Step 14. Attach syringe and blood collection tubes to the blood transfer device and fill tubes in the correct order.

Step 15. After tubes are filled, mix immediately by gentle inversion for the appropriate number of inversions.

Step 16. Label all tubes in front of the patient and confirm with the patient or identification band that the information is correct.

Step 17. Scrub the hub for 15 seconds with alcohol to remove blood.

Step 18. Attach prefilled nonsterile 10-mL saline syringe and flush. Use two syringes for a total of 20 mL. If there are lumens that are not being used, flush each of those lumens with 10 mL of saline.

Step 19. Resume previous fluids, if applicable.

Step 20. Prepare sample and requisition form for transport to the laboratory.

Step 21. Dispose of used supplies in biohazard container.

Step 22. Remove gloves, sanitize hands, and thank the patient.

PROCEDURE 8-3 Blood Sample Collection From a Central Venous Access Device (Continued)

 SAFETY TIP 8-4

Proper hand hygiene should be followed, especially when manipulating a central line catheter because most catheters are placed into large vasculature in and around the heart.

 TECHNICAL TIP 8-7

Sterile gloves are not required when collecting blood for laboratory testing.

 TECHNICAL TIP 8-6

Procedures for the various types of central line catheters vary slightly and should be performed following the correct flush protocol according to facility policy.

PROCEDURE 8-4 Blood Collection From an Implanted Port

EQUIPMENT:

Sterile drape
Sterile gloves
Noncoring needle,
Two 10-mL syringes
Two 10-mL flush syringes filled with saline
One 10-mL syringe filled with heparinized
    flush solution (follow institutional protocol)
Chlorhexidine gluconate sponge or alcohol
    and iodine pads
One 5-mL syringe

2 × 2 gauze pads
Dressing to cover insertion site

 SAFETY TIP 8-5

Sterile gloves are worn when accessing ports. Sterile technique is maintained throughout the procedure.

PROCEDURE:

Step 1. Identify the patient verbally by having him or her state both the first name and last name, and date of birth. Compare the information on the patient's ID band with the requisition form.

Step 2. Explain the procedure and obtain the patient consent.

Step 3. Sanitize hands and put on gloves.

PROCEDURE 8-4   Blood Collection From an Implanted Port (Continued)

Step 4. Palpate the shoulder area to locate and identify the septum of the access port.

Step 5. Prep the area with a vigorous scrub using a chlorhexidine gluconate applicator. If using alcohol and iodine pads, prep a circular motion from within to outward, approximately 4 to 6 inches, first with the alcohol pad and then with the iodine swab. Allow iodine to dry completely (30–60 seconds).

Step 6. Connect the noncoring needle tubing on the end of one 10-mL saline flush syringe and prime the needle with saline until it is expelled.

Step 7. Locate the septum of the port with the nondominant hand; firmly anchor the port between the thumb and the forefinger.

Step 8. Holding the noncoring needle with the other hand, puncture the skin and insert the needle at a 90-degree angle into the septum using firm pressure. Advance the needle until resistance is met and the needle touches the back wall of the port.

Step 9. Inject 1 to 2 mL of saline, observe the area for swelling and ease of flow; if swelling occurs, reposition the needle in the port without withdrawing it from the skin. If there is not swelling, aspirate for blood return. If blood return is observed, continue to flush with saline.

Step 10. Using the same syringe, aspirate 10 mL of blood and discard it. If samples will be collected for coagulation studies, discard 20 mL.

Step 11. Attach the syringe or the evacuated tube holder to the needle tubing and collect the minimum blood necessary for ordered laboratory tests.

Step 12. Dispense the blood into the appropriate blood collection tubes using a blood transfer device if a syringe is used in the correct order of fill. Mix the blood by gentle inversion three to eight times.

Step 13. Flush the needle and the port with 20 mL of saline.

Step 14. Change syringes and flush with 3 mL of heparinized saline or according to your facility's policy.

Step 15. Remove the needle and apply a sterile dressing over site.

Step 16. Label samples appropriately, and confirm label with patient or identification band.

Step 17. Remove gloves and sanitize hands.

Step 18. Prepare sample and requisition form for transport to the laboratory.

Step 19. Dispose of used supplies in appropriate biohazard containers.

Step 20. Thank the patient.

 TECHNICAL TIP 8-8

Proficiency in the care of catheters will result with continued practice of technique and skills.

BIBLIOGRAPHY

Infusion Nursing Standards of Practice: *J Infusion Nurs* 34(Suppl. 1), 2011.

Methodist Hospital Nursing Service Policy and Procedure Manual: Blood Specimen Collection From Vascular Access Device. Omaha, NE, Methodist Hospital, 2014.

INTERNET RESOURCES

www.journalofinfusionnursing.com

Seattle treatment education project. The body. Available at http://www.thebody.com/content/art1786.html?ts=pf Accessed 8/30/2008.

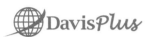 For additional material, please visit http://davisplus.fadavis.com.

REVIEW QUESTIONS

1. **When collecting blood samples after inserting a peripheral IV catheter, the:**
   a. Line should be flushed before the blood is collected
   b. Line should be flushed after the blood is collected
   c. Catheter tubing should be taped to the patient first
   d. Tourniquet should not be removed

2. **Which of the following is a tunneled catheter?**
   a. Midline peripheral catheter
   b. PICC line
   c. Hickman
   d. Peripheral IV

3. **Blood collected from CVCs is collected in evacuated tubes by attaching a/an:**
   a. Sterile 20-gauge needle to the collection syringe
   b. Evacuated tube holder to the catheter line
   c. Blood transfer device to the collection syringe
   d. Luer-Lock to the catheter line

4. **Evacuated tubes containing blood collected from a CVC should be gently mixed:**
   a. After the line has been flushed
   b. As soon as they are filled
   c. After they are labeled
   d. As soon as the port has been heparinized

5. **Blood cannot be drawn from which of the following catheters?**
   a. Midline peripheral
   b. Groshong
   c. PICC line
   d. Hickman

6. **What should the blood collector observe when flushing the IV tubing?**
   a. Swelling or pain in the area
   b. Ease of injecting flush solution into the catheter
   c. Ability to obtain blood back into the flush syringe
   d. All of the above

7. **Blood cannot be drawn from a PICC line that is infusing:**
   a. Antibiotics
   b. Total parental nutrition
   c. Dextrose
   d. Pain medication

8. **A tourniquet should not be applied when collecting blood using a/an:**
   a. Peripheral IV catheter
   b. Hickman catheter
   c. PICC line
   d. Implanted port

9. **Blood collected from which of the following catheters does not require a waste tube?**
   a. Peripheral IV line
   b. PICC line
   c. Groshong
   d. Hickman

10. **Which of the following has a self-sealing septum that is accessed with a noncoring needle?**
    a. Implanted port
    b. PICC
    c. Hickman
    d. Peripheral IV

FOR FURTHER STUDY

1. State two ways in which blood collected after insertion of a peripheral IV could be hemolyzed.

2. Explain the purpose of flush syringes.

3. What additional precaution must be taken when coagulation tests are drawn from CVCs?

4. Why is specialized training required for personnel collecting samples from CVCs?

CASE STUDY 8-1

Mr. Smith, diagnosed with pneumonia, was in the hospital for several days and required multiple blood collections throughout the day. He also was receiving antibiotics by IV. After many venipunctures, it was very difficult to find a good vein that was not covered by hematomas. A PICC line was placed in Mr. Smith for blood collection and medication infusion. The doctor ordered an APTT, CBC, and basic metabolic panel every 4 hours.

1. What must the nurse do before collecting the sample?

2. How many and what size syringes are needed?

3. How will the blood be placed in the collection tubes?

4. What is the correct order of fill?

CASE STUDY 8-2

Blood was collected from Mrs. Artz's CVAD for an antifactor X assay to monitor her unfractionated heparin level. The result was markedly higher than the previous result and the therapeutic range. Blood was re-collected from a peripheral vein for the antifactor X assay and the value was within the therapeutic range.

1. What could have caused this discrepancy?

2. What two substances are used to flush an IV or catheter?

3. What is the flush protocol when using one of the above substances?

4. What volume of blood should be discarded or used before drawing coagulation tests?

EVALUATION OF PERIPHERAL IV INSERTION

RATING SYSTEM

2 = *Satisfactorily*

1 = *Needs improvement*

0 = *Incorrect/did not perform*

NAME: _____

Prior to entering patient's room:

_____ 1. Checks IV fluid for correct name, expiration date, contamination, and leaks.

_____ 2. Spikes bag.

_____ 3. Fills drip chamber and primes tubing (free of air bubbles).

Enters patient's room:

_____ 4. Introduces self, establishes rapport.

_____ 5. Identifies patient.

_____ 6. Assesses patient history (specifically for allergies).

_____ 7. Explains procedure to patient.

_____ 8. Prepares the environment: privacy, lighting, and bed adjustment.

_____ 9. Prepares equipment.

_____ 10. Sanitizes hands and puts on gloves.

_____ 11. Applies tourniquet 4 to 6 inches above puncture site.

_____ 12. Palpates for suitable vein, releases tourniquet.

_____ 13. Cleanses puncture site appropriately.

_____ 14. Reties tourniquet.

_____ 15. Stabilizes vein and inserts IV catheter watching for flashback.

_____ 16. Releases tourniquet.

_____ 17. Advances catheter into vein.

_____ 18. Occludes vein proximal to catheter.

_____ 19. Removes needle, activates needle safety device, and disposes of it into proper sharps container.

_____ 20. Attaches IV tubing to catheter.

_____ 21. Opens clamp, runs IV to ensure patent line, watches for signs of infiltration.

_____ 22. Adjusts clamp for correct IV flow per situation.

_____ 23. Applies sterile dressing to IV site.

_____ 24. Secures IV with tape or other device.

_____ 25. Explains precautions and ambulation procedure to patient.

_____ 26. Maintains aseptic technique and adheres to standard precautions throughout procedure.

TOTAL POINTS _____

MAXIMUM POINTS = 52

COMMENTS:

EVALUATION OF BLOOD SAMPLE COLLECTION FROM CENTRAL VENOUS ACCESS DEVICE

RATING SYSTEM

2 = Satisfactory

1 = Needs Improvement

0 = Incorrect/Did Not Perform

NAME: _____

_____ 1. Examines requisition and verifies patient using two identifiers according to normal protocol.

_____ 2. Explains the procedure and obtains patient's consent.

_____ 3. Correctly assembles equipment.

_____ 4. Positions the patient in a supine position.

_____ 5. Sanitizes hands.

_____ 6. Puts on gloves.

_____ 7. Discontinues administration of all infusates into the CVAD.

_____ 8. Chooses the proximal lumen to obtain the sample.

_____ 9. Disinfects the injection cap with an alcohol wipe using a friction scrub for the correct amount of time.

_____ 10. Flushes with 10 mL normal saline or 20 mL of saline if TPN or heparin was infusing.

_____ 11. Uses same syringe and aspirates 5 mL blood.

_____ 12. Removes syringe and discards it in biohazard container.

_____ 13. Waits 10 to 15 seconds to draw sample.

_____ 14. Uses sterile syringe to collect the smallest amount of blood required.

_____ 15. Connects a blood transfer device to the collection syringe and fills evacuated tubes completely and according to the correct order of fill.

_____ 16. Immediately mixes the tubes by gentle inversion three to eight times depending on the tube.

_____ 17. Labels each tube correctly and confirms identification with patient or patient's identification band.

_____ 18. Attaches prefilled nonsterile 10-mL saline syringe and flush and flushes using two syringes for a total of 20 mL.

_____ 19. Resumes infusions in all lumens.

_____ 20. Prepares sample and requisitions forms for transport to the laboratory.

_____ 21. Disposes of used supplies in biohazard container.

_____ 22. Removes gloves, sanitizes hands, and thanks the patient.

TOTAL POINTS

MAXIMUM POINTS = 44

COMMENTS:

EVALUATION OF BLOOD SAMPLE COLLECTION FROM IMPLANTED PORT

RATING SYSTEM

2 = Satisfactory

1 = Needs Improvement

0 = Incorrect/Did Not Perform

NAME: _____

_____ 1. Examines requisition and verifies patient using two identifiers according to normal protocol.

_____ 2. Explains procedure and obtains consent.

_____ 3. Sanitizes hands and puts on gloves.

_____ 4. Correctly assembles equipment.

_____ 5. Palpates the shoulder area locating the septum of the access port.

_____ 6. Preps the area with a vigorous scrub using chlorhexidine gluconate applicator.

_____ 7. Connects the noncoring needle tubing to the end of a 10-mL saline flush syringe and primes the needle with saline.

_____ 8. Anchors the port between the thumb and the forefinger with the nondominant hand.

_____ 9. Hold the noncoring needle with the dominant hand and inserts the needle at a 90-degree angle into the septum.

_____ 10. Advances the needle until resistance is met.

_____ 11. Inject 1 to 2 mL of saline observing for swelling. Aspirates for blood return if there is no swelling. Continues to flush with saline.

_____ 12. Uses same syringe and aspirates 10 mL of blood and discards it. Discards 20 mL for coagulation tests.

_____ 13. Attaches syringe or evacuated tube holder to the needle tubing and collects the minimum blood necessary for laboratory tests in the correct order of draw.

_____ 14. Dispenses blood into correct blood collection tubes using a blood transfer device when using a syringe.

_____ 15. Mixes blood by gentle inversion three to eight times.

_____ 16. Flushes the needle and port with 20 mL of saline.

_____ 17. Removes needle and applies sterile dressing over site.

_____ 18. Labels tubes and confirms the information with patient or identification band.

_____ 19. Removes gloves and sanitizes hands.

_____ 20. Prepares sample and requisition form for transport to the laboratory.

_____ 21. Disposes of used supplies in appropriate biohazard containers.

_____ 22. Thanks the patient.

TOTAL POINTS

MAXIMUM POINT 44

COMMENTS:

A

Laboratory Tests and the Required Type of Anticoagulants and Volume of Blood

Test	Collection Tube	Comments	Dept.	Clinical Correlation
Acid phosphatase	Serum (red or gold) or plasma (green) gel barrier tube	Freeze serum	C	Prostate cancer
Adrenocorticotropic hormone (ACTH)	Lavender, siliconized glass or plastic	Freeze plasma	C	Adrenal and pituitary gland function
Alanine aminotransferase (ALT)	Plasma (green) or serum (red or gold) gel barrier tube		C	Liver disorders
Albumin	Serum (red or gold) or plasma (green) gel barrier tube		C	Malnutrition or liver disorders
Alcohol	Red or gray or lavender		C	Intoxication
Aldosterone	Red	Patient should be lying down for at least 30 minutes prior to blood collection.	C	Adrenal function

Continued

Test	Collection Tube	Comments	Dept.	Clinical Correlation
Alkaline phosphatase (ALP)	Serum (red or gold) or plasma (green) gel barrier tube		C	Bone disorders
Aluminum	Royal blue with ethylenediaminetetraacetic acid (EDTA)		C	Toxicity
Ammonia (NH$_3$)	Lavender or green	Send on ice slurry	C	Hepatic encephalopathy
Amylase	Serum (red or gold) gel barrier tube		C	Pancreatitis
Antibiotic assay (amikacin, gentamicin, theophylline, tobramycin, vancomycin)	Red; clear nongel Microtainer	No gel barrier tubes	C	Broad-spectrum antibiotics
Antibody ID/screen	Lavender or pink	Blood bank ID	BB	Blood transfusion
Antidiuretic hormone (ADH)	Lavender	Freeze plasma	C	Pituitary function
Anti-hepatitis A virus	Serum (red or gold); red		C	Viral hepatitis A infection
Anti-hepatitis C virus	Serum (red or gold) gel barrier tube; red		S	Viral hepatitis C infection
Anti-HIV	Red		S	HIV
Antinuclear antibody (ANA)	Serum (red or gold) gel barrier tube; red		S	Systemic lupus erythematosus/ autoimmune disorders
Antistreptolysin O (ASO) titer	Red	Refrigerate immediately	S	Rheumatic fever
Antithrombin III	Light blue		CO	Coagulation disorders
Apo-A, Apo-B lipoprotein	Serum (red or gold) gel barrier tube		C	Cardiac risk
Aspartate aminotransferase (AST)	Plasma (green) or serum (red or gold) gel barrier tube		C	Liver disorders, cardiac muscle damage
Basic metabolic panel (BMP)	Plasma (green) or serum (red or gold) gel barrier tube		C	Metabolism
Beta human chorionic gonadotropin (Beta HCG)	Plasma (green) or serum (red or gold) gel barrier tube		C	Pregnancy, testicular cancer
Blood culture	Blood culture bottles (two bottles, aerobic and anaerobic, two yellow sodium polyanethol sulfonate [SPS] tubes)	Aseptic technique	M	Septicemia
Blood group and type (ABO and Rh)	Lavender or pink	Blood bank ID	BB	ABO group and Rh factor
Blood urea nitrogen (BUN)	Plasma (green) or serum (red or gold) gel barrier tube		C	Kidney disorders

Test	Collection Tube	Comments	Dept.	Clinical Correlation
Bilirubin, total and direct (Bili)	Plasma (green) or serum (red or gold) gel barrier tube; amber or green Microtainer	Protect from light	C	Liver disorders and hemolytic disorders
Brain natriuretic peptide (BNP)	Lavender; white plasma preparation tube, serum gel barrier tube	Stable for 4 hours	C	Congestive heart failure
Calcium	Plasma (green) or serum (red or gold) gel barrier tube	Deliver immediately	C	Bone disorders
C-reactive protein (CRP)	Serum (red or gold) gel barrier tube		C	Inflammatory disorders
Chemistry panels (renal, hepatic, cardiac, comprehensive, metabolic)	Plasma (green) or serum (red or gold) gel barrier tube		C	Evaluates various organ systems
Cholesterol	Plasma (green) or serum (red or gold) gel barrier tube		C	Coronary artery disease
Cold agglutinins	Red	Must be kept at 37°C; no gel tube	S	Atypical pneumonia
Complement levels	Serum (red or gold) gel barrier tube		C	Immune system function/ autoimmune disorders
Complete blood count (CBC)	Lavender		H	Anemia, infection, leukemia, or bleeding disorders
Copper	Serum royal blue		C	Biliary cirrhosis
Cortisol	Serum (red or gold) gel barrier tube; red	Serum only Timed specimen (a.m.)	C	Adrenal cortex function
Creatine kinase (CK)	Plasma (green) or serum (red or gold) gel barrier tube		C	Myocardial infarction, muscle damage
Creatine kinase isoenzymes (CK-MB, CK-MM, CK-BB)	Plasma (green) or serum (red or gold) gel barrier tube		C	Myocardial infarction, muscle damage, brain damage
Creatinine	Plasma (green) or serum (red or gold) gel barrier tube		C	Kidney disorders
C-reactive protein	Red or serum (red or gold) gel barrier tube		C	Inflammatory processes
Crossmatch	Lavender; pink	Blood bank ID band remains on 72 hours	BB	Blood compatibility
Digoxin	Plasma (green) or serum (red or gold) gel barrier tube; red		C	Heart stimulant
D-Dimer (D-DI)	Light blue	Tube must be full (stable for 4 hours)	CO	DIC and thrombotic disorders
Direct anti-human globulin test (DAT) or direct Coombs	Lavender		BB	Anemia or hemolytic disease of the newborn
Disseminated intravascular coagulation panel (DIC)	Light blue		CO	Coagulation/fibrinolytic systems

Continued

Test	Collection Tube	Comments	Dept.	Clinical Correlation
Drug screen	Red	No gel		Detection and identification of drugs
Electrolytes (Lytes)	Plasma (green) or serum (red or gold) gel barrier tube		C	Fluid and acid–base balance
Erythrocyte sedimentation rate (ESR)	Lavender		H	Inflammatory disorders
Ethanol/alcohol (ETOH)	Gray	Do not open tube until testing; may require chain of custody	C	Intoxication
Factor assays	Light blue	Tube must be full	C	Detect specific factor function
Febrile antibody panel	Red		S	Antibody screen for *Salmonella, Rickettsia, Brucella, Francisella tularensis*
Ferritin	Serum (red or gold) or plasma (green) gel barrier tube		C	Iron deficiency
Fibrin degradation products (FDP)	Special light blue tube with thrombin	Tube will only fill to 2 mL and should clot immediately	CO	Disseminated intravascular coagulation
Fibrinogen	Light blue	Tube must be full	C	Coagulation disorders
Fluorescent antinuclear antibody (FANA)	Serum (red or gold) gel barrier tube; red		S	Systemic lupus erythematosus/ autoimmune disorders
Fluorescent treponemal antibody-absorbed (FTA-ABS)	Serum (red or gold) gel barrier tube; red		S	Syphilis
Folate	Serum (red or gold) gel barrier tube; red		C	Anemia
Gamma-glutamyl transpeptidase (GGT)	Serum (red or gold) gel barrier tube; Red		C	Liver disease
Gastrin	Serum (red or gold) gel barrier tube	Transport in ice slurry	C	Gastric malignancy or pernicious anemia
Glucose (FBS)	Plasma (green) or serum (red or gold) gel barrier tube; red; gray		C	Hypoglycemia or diabetes mellitus
Hematocrit	Lavender		H	Anemia
Hemoglobin	Lavender		H	Anemia
Hemoglobin A_{1C}	Lavender		C	Diabetes mellitus
Hemoglobin electrophoresis	Lavender		C	Hemoglobin abnormalities
Hemoglobin/hematocrit (H&H); Hgb/Hct	Lavender		H	Anemia
Heparin Anti-Xa Assay	Light blue tube		CO	Heparin therapy
Hepatitis B core antibody	Serum (red or gold) gel barrier tube; red		S	Past or present hepatitis B infection

Test	Collection Tube	Comments	Dept.	Clinical Correlation
Hepatitis B surface antibody	Serum (red or gold) gel barrier tube; red		S	Immunity to hepatitis B
Hepatitis B surface antigen	Serum (red or gold) gel barrier tube; red		S	Hepatitis B infection
Human chorionic gonadotropin (Beta HCG)	Plasma (green) or serum (red or gold) gel barrier tube		C	Pregnancy, testicular tumor
INR/PT	Light blue	Tube must be full	C	Coumadin therapy
Immunoglobulin levels	Red; plasma (green) or serum (red or gold) gel barrier tube		C	Immune system function
Insulin	Serum (red or gold) gel barrier tube		C	Glucose metabolism and pancreatic function
Ionized calcium (iCa^{2+})	Serum (red or gold) gel barrier tube; red; arterial blood gas syringe	Tube must be full; may use arterial blood gas syringe	C	Follow-up test for abnormal total calcium results
Iron	Plasma (green) or serum (red or gold) gel barrier tube		C	Anemia
Iron-binding capacity	Plasma (green or serum (red or gold) gel barrier tube		C	Anemia
Lactate dehydrogenase (LD)	Plasma (green) or serum (red or gold) gel barrier tube		C	Myocardial infarction
Lactate (lactic acid) (Lact)	Plasma (green) gel barrier tube; gray; arterial blood gas syringe	Send in ice slurry; analyze in 15 minutes Draw without tourniquet	C	Muscle disorders
Lead (Pb)	Royal blue EDTA; tan EDTA; lavender Microtainer		C	Neurological function
Lipase	Plasma (green) or serum (red or gold) gel barrier tube; red		C	Pancreatitis
Lipoproteins (high-density lipoprotein [HDL], low-density lipoprotein [LDL], very low-density lipoprotein [VLDL])	Plasma (green) or serum (red or gold) gel barrier tube		C	Coronary risk
Lithium (Li)	Serum (red or gold) gel barrier tube; red	Draw 12 hours post-dose	C	Antidepressant drug monitoring
Magnesium	Serum (red or gold) gel barrier tube; red		C	Musculoskeletal disorders
MI panel (myoglobin, creatine kinase isoenzyme (CK-MB), troponin)	Plasma (green) gel barrier tube; white plasma preparation tube	Stable 4 hours; EDTA plasma from a lavender stopper tube or a white PPT	C	Myocardial infarction
Mononucleosis screen (Mono test)	Serum (red or gold) gel barrier tube; red		S	Infectious mononucleosis
Myoglobin	Serum (red or gold) gel barrier tube; red		C	Muscle damage

Continued

Test	Collection Tube	Comments	Dept.	Clinical Correlation
Osmolality	Serum (red or gold) gel barrier tube; red		C	Comatose patients
pH	Green; nongel	Send on ice slurry	C	Acid–base balance
Parathyroid hormone (PTH)	Lavender		C	Parathyroid function
Partial thromboplastin time (PTT); activated partial thromboplastin time (APTT)	Light blue	Full tube; nonheparinized samples are stable at RT up to 4 hours; heparinized samples must be centrifuged within 1 hour and are stable up to 4 hours	CO	Heparin therapy and coagulation disorders
Phosphorus	Plasma (green) or serum (red or gold) gel barrier tube		C	Endocrine and bone disorders
Platelet aggregation	Light blue and lavender		C	Platelet function
Platelet (Plt)	Lavender		H	Bleeding disorders
Potassium	Plasma (green) or serum (red or gold) gel barrier tube; red		C	Muscle function, heart contraction/cardiac output
Prostate-specific antigen (PSA)	Serum (red or gold) gel barrier tube		C	Prostatic cancer
Prostatic acid phosphatase (PAP)	Serum (red or gold) gel barrier tube		C	Prostatic cancer
Protein	Serum (red or gold) gel barrier tube		C	Liver, kidney, bone marrow, metabolic, or nutritional disorders
Protein electrophoresis	Serum (red or gold) gel barrier tube; red		C	Multiple myeloma/ abnormal proteins
Prothrombin time (PT)	Light blue	Full tube; stable at RT up to 24 hours	CO	Coumadin therapy and coagulation disorders
Quant proteins (C3, C4, IgG, IgA, IgM), haptoglobin	Plasma (green) or serum (red or gold) gel barrier tube; red		S	Immunoglobulin disorders, hemolytic anemia
Red blood cell count	Lavender		H	Anemia
Reticulocyte count (Retic)	Lavender		H	Bone marrow function
Rheumatoid factor	Serum (red or gold) gel barrier tube; red		S	Rheumatoid arthritis
Rubella titer	Serum (red or gold) gel barrier tube; red		S	Immunity to German measles
Sickle cell screening	Lavender		H	Sickle cell anemia
Sodium	Plasma (green) or serum (red or gold) gel barrier tube		C	Acid–base balance
T-cell count	Lavender		S	Immune function/HIV monitoring

Test	Collection Tube	Comments	Dept.	Clinical Correlation
Testosterone	Serum (red or gold) gel barrier tube		C	Testicular function
Therapeutic drugs (digoxin, theophylline [theo], phenobarbital, phenytoin [Pheny], carbamazepine [Carb], valproic acid [val ac])	Red; clear nongel Microtainer	No gel barrier; centrifuge and separate within 1 hour	C	Monitor medications for seizures, bipolar disorders, epilepsy, asthma
Thyroid-stimulating hormone/Free T4 (TSH/T4)	Plasma (green) or serum (red or gold) gel barrier tube		C	Thyroid conditions
Total protein (TP)	Serum (red or gold) gel barrier tube		C	Kidney and liver disorders
Triglycerides	Plasma (green) or serum (red or gold) gel barrier tube		C	Coronary heart disease
Troponin I and T	Serum (red or gold) gel barrier tube; lavender; white plasma preparation tube		C	Myocardial function
Type and screen	Lavender/pink	Blood bank ID band	BB	Blood transfusion
Uric acid	Serum (red or gold) gel barrier tube		C	Kidney disorders, gout
Venereal Disease Research Laboratory (VDRL)	Serum (red or gold) gel barrier tube; red		S	Syphilis
Viral load	Lavender; white plasma preparation tube; serum (red or gold) gel barrier tube	Freeze plasma immediately	S	HIV monitoring
Vitamin B_{12}	Plasma (green) or serum (red or gold) gel barrier tube; red	Protect from light	C	Anemia
Vitamin D	Serum (red or gold) gel barrier tube		C	Calcium absorption
Western blot	Red		S	Human immunodeficiency virus
White blood cell count (WBC)	Lavender		H	Infection or leukemia
Zinc	Plain royal blue tube		C	Zinc deficiency

Laboratory department codes: BB = blood bank; C = chemistry; CO = coagulation; H = hematology; ID = identification; M = microbiology; RT = room temperature; S = serology.

*Follow evacuated tubes manufacturer's instructions when using gel barrier tubes for serology tests.

Modified with permission from Strasinger, S.K., and Di Lorenzo, M.S.: The Phlebotomy Textbook, ed. 3. Philadelphia, F.A. Davis, 2011.

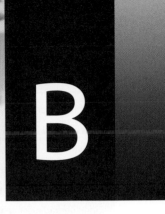

Clinical Correlations of Blood Tests Related to Body Systems

Test	Clinical Correlation
Circulatory System	
Activated clotting time (ACT)	Heparin therapy
Activated partial thromboplastin time [APTT (PTT)]	Heparin therapy or coagulation disorders
Antibody (Ab) screen	Blood transfusion
Antistreptolysin O (ASO) titer	Rheumatic fever
Antithrombin III	Coagulation disorders
Apo-A, Apo-B lipoprotein	Cardiac risk
Arterial blood gases	Acid–base balance
Aspartate aminotransferase (AST)	Cardiac muscle damage
Bilirubin	Hemolytic disorders
Blood culture	Septicemia
Blood group and type	ABO group and Rh factor
Brain natriuretic peptide (BNP)	Congestive heart failure
C-reactive protein (CRP)	Inflammatory disorders
Cholesterol	Coronary artery disease

Continued

Test	Clinical Correlation
Complete blood count (CBC)	Anemia, infection, leukemia, or bleeding disorders
Creatine kinase (CK)	Myocardial infarction
Creatine kinase isoenzymes (CK-MB)	Myocardial infarction
Disseminated intravascular coagulation (DIC) panel	Coagulation/fibrinolytic systems
Digoxin	Heart stimulant
Direct anti–human globulin test (DAT) or direct Coombs	Anemia or hemolytic disease of the newborn
Erythrocyte sedimentation rate (ESR)	Inflammatory disorders
Fibrin degradation products (FDP)	Disseminated intravascular coagulation
Fibrinogen	Coagulation disorders
Folate	Anemia
Hematocrit (Hct)	Anemia
Hemoglobin (Hgb)	Anemia
Hemoglobin (Hgb) electrophoresis	Hemoglobin abnormalities
Heparin Anti-Xa Assay	Heparin therapy
High-density lipoprotein (HDL)	Coronary risk
Iron	Anemia
Lactate dehydrogenase (LD)	Myocardial infarction
Low-density lipoprotein (LDL)	Coronary risk
Myoglobin	Myocardial infarction
Platelet (Plt) count	Bleeding tendencies
Platelet aggregation	Platelet function
Potassium	Heart contraction/cardiac output
Prothrombin time (PT)	Coumadin therapy and coagulation disorders
Reticulocyte (Retic) count	Bone marrow function
Sickle cell screening	Sickle cell anemia
Total iron binding capacity (TIBC)	Anemia
Triglycerides	Coronary artery disease
Troponin I and T	Myocardial infarction
Type and crossmatch (T & C)	Blood transfusion
Type and screen	Blood transfusion
White blood cell (WBC) count	Infections or leukemia
Vitamin B_{12}	Anemia

Lymphatic System

Test	Clinical Correlation
Anti-HIV	HIV screening test
Antinuclear antibody (ANA)	Systemic lupus erythematosus/autoimmune disorders
Complete blood count (CBC)	Infectious mononucleosis
Complement levels	Immune system function/autoimmune disorders
Fluorescent antinuclear antibody (FANA)	Systemic lupus erythematosus/autoimmune disorders

Test	Clinical Correlation
Immunoglobulin (Ig) levels	Immune system function
Monospot	Infectious mononucleosis
p24 antigen	HIV
Protein electrophoresis	Multiple myeloma
T-cell count	Immune function/HIV monitoring
Viral load	HIV monitoring
Western blot	HIV confirmation test

Skeletal System

Test	Clinical Correlation
Alkaline phosphatase (ALP)	Bone disorders
Antinuclear antibody (ANA)	Systemic lupus erythematosus/collagen disorders
Calcium (Ca)	Bone disorders
Erythrocyte sedimentation rate (ESR)	Inflammation
Fluorescent antinuclear antibody (FANA)	Systemic lupus erythematosus/collagen disorders
Phosphorus (P)	Skeletal disorders
Rheumatoid factor (RF)	Rheumatoid arthritis
Uric acid	Gout
Vitamin D	Calcium absorption

Muscular System

Test	Clinical Correlation
Creatine kinase (CK)	Muscle damage
Creatine kinase isoenzymes (CK-MB)	Muscle damage
Lactic acid	Muscle disorders
Magnesium (Mg)	Musculoskeletal disorders
Myoglobin	Muscle damage
Potassium (K)	Muscle function

Nervous System

Test	Clinical Correlation
Creatine kinase isoenzymes	Brain damage
Cerebrospsinal fluid (CSF) analysis (cell count/differential, glucose, protein, culture and gram stain)	Neurological disorders or meningitis
Drug screening	Therapeutic drug monitoring or drug abuse
Lead	Neurological function
Lithium (Li)	Antidepressant drug monitoring

Respiratory System

Test	Clinical Correlation
Arterial blood gases (ABGs)	Acid–base balance
Cold agglutinins	Atypical pneumonia
Complete blood count (CBC)	Pneumonia
Electrolytes (Lytes)	Acid–base balance
Gram stain	Microbial infection
Throat and sputum cultures	Bacterial infection

Continued

Test	Clinical Correlation
Digestive System	
Alanine aminotransferase (ALT)	Liver disorders
Albumin	Malnutrition or liver disorders
Alcohol	Intoxication/liver function
Alkaline phosphatase (ALP)	Liver disorders
Ammonia	Severe liver disorders
Amylase	Pancreatitis
Anti–hepatitis A virus (anti-HAV)	Viral hepatitis
Anti–hepatitis C virus (anti-HCV)	Viral hepatitis
Aspartate aminotransferase (AST)	Liver disorders
Bilirubin	Liver disorders
Carcinoembryonic antigen (CEA)	Carcinoma detection and monitoring
Complete blood count (CBC)	Appendicitis, peritonitis, or other infection
Gamma-glutamyl transferase (GGT)	Early liver disorders
Gastrin	Gastric malignancy
Hepatitis A, B, and C immunoassays	Hepatitis A, B, and C screening
Hepatitis B core antibody	Past or present hepatitis B infection
Hepatitis B surface antibody	Hepatitis B immunity
Hepatitis B surface antigen	Active hepatitis B infection
Lactate dehydrogenase (LD)	Liver disorders
Lipase	Pancreatitis
Occult blood	Gastrointestinal bleeding or intestinal malignancy
Stool culture	Pathogenic bacteria
Total protein (TP)	Liver disorders
Urinary System	
Albumin	Kidney disorders
Ammonia	Kidney function
Antistreptolysin O (ASO) titer	Acute glomerulonephritis
Blood urea nitrogen (BUN)	Kidney disorders
Creatinine	Kidney disorders
Creatinine clearance	Glomerular filtration
Electrolytes (Lytes)	Fluid and electrolyte balance
Osmolality	Fluid and electrolyte balance
Routine urinalysis (UA)	Renal or metabolic disorders
Total protein (TP)	Kidney disorders
Uric acid	Kidney disorders
Urine culture	Bacterial infection

Test	Clinical Correlation
Endocrine System	
Adrenocorticotropic hormone (ACTH)	Adrenal and pituitary gland function
Aldosterone	Adrenal function
Antidiuretic hormone (ADH)	Pituitary function
Calcium (Ca)	Parathyroid function
Catecholamines	Adrenal function
Cortisol	Adrenal cortex function
Glucose	Hypoglycemia or diabetes mellitus
Glucose tolerance test (GTT)	Hypoglycemia or diabetes mellitus
Growth hormone (GH)	Pituitary gland function
Insulin	Glucose metabolism and pancreatic function
Parathyroid hormone (PTH)	Parathyroid function
Phosphorus (P)	Endocrine disorders
Testosterone	Testicular function
Thyroid function (T_3, T_4, TSH) panel	Thyroid function
Reproductive System	
Estradiol, estriol, and estrogen	Ovarian or placental function
Fluorescent treponemal antibody–absorbed (FTA-ABS)	Syphilis
Genital culture	Microbial infection
Gram stain	Microbial infection
Human chorionic gonadotropin (Beta HCG)	Pregnancy
Pap smear (Pap)	Cervical or vaginal carcinoma
Prostate-specific antigen (PSA)	Prostatic cancer
Prostatic acid phosphatase (PAP)	Prostatic cancer
Rapid plasma reagin (RPR)	Syphilis
Rubella titer	Immunity to German measles
Semen analysis	Infertility or effectiveness of vasectomy
Toxoplasma antibody screening	Toxoplasma infection
Vaginal wet prep	Fungal infection
Venereal Disease Research Laboratory (VDRL)	Syphilis

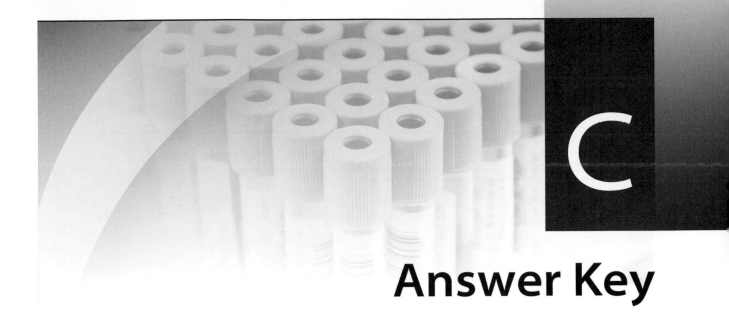

Answer Key

CHAPTER 1

Review Questions

1. C
2. B
3. D
4. B
5. C
6. B
7. B
8. C
9. A
10. B

For Further Study

1. The CLIA is a governmental regulatory agency administered by the Centers for Medicare & Medicaid Services and the Food and Drug Administration that determines the requirements for persons performing waived, provider-performed microscopy procedures (PPMP), moderate-complexity, and high-complexity testing.
2. a. Hand hygiene
   b. Portal of entry
   c. Portal of exit
3. a. Standard precautions: Not wearing gloves for each patient or not changing gloves between patients.

b. HIPAA: Leaking confidential information concerning a patient.
   c. OSHA Bloodborne Pathogen Standard: Not activating safety devices on needles after use.
   d. Postexposure prophylaxis: Exposure to blood through a needlestick.

Case Study 1-1

1. Clean the site and report it to her supervisor.
2. Following the correct one-handed procedure for activating the safety shield over the needle.
3. The blood collector is counseled about receiving PEP using zidovudine or other anti-HIV medications. Medications are started within 24 hours. The blood collector is retested at intervals of 6 weeks, 12 weeks, and 6 months.

Case Study 1-2

1. The sample must be centrifuged at the manufacturer's requirements for the speed and times of centrifugation. Tubes must be balanced in the centrifuge. Serum samples must be fully clotted (usually for 30 minutes) before centrifugation. Plasma samples may be centrifuged immediately after the sample has been well mixed following collection. Plasma and serum must be removed from the cells within 2 hours.
2. Carefully using a disposable pipette to transfer a specimen to a correctly labeled aliquot tube.

3. Samples are packaged and shipped according to the U.S. Department of Transportation. Samples should be placed in closed, leakproof primary containers and enclosed in a secondary leakproof container with sufficient absorbent material.

CHAPTER 2

Review Questions

1. D
2. D
3. C
4. B
5. A
6. C
7. B
8. A
9. B
10. B

For Further Study

1. No, because EDTA interferes with factor V and the thrombin-fibrinogen reaction.
2. The sample was hemolyzed during the blood transfer process.
3. The SST contains a serum separator gel to prevent cellular contamination.
4. Plasma. This fluid does contain fibrinogen.

Case Study 2-1

1. The CBC should be collected in a lavender stopper tube. The electrolytes should be collected in a green gel separator tube (PST).
2. Green gel separator tube (PST) and then lavender.
3. a. The sample was hemolyzed because a 25-gauge needle was used causing increased plasma potassium levels.
   b. The sample was too vigorously mixed after collection causing hemolyis and increased potassium levels.

Case Study 2-2

1. The tubes were not filled to the correct amount. It must be a 9:1 ratio of blood to anticoagulant.
2. There is 0.5 mL of air in the tubing of a winged blood collection set. The air in the line caused the tube to not fill to the correct level.

3. A discard tube should have been used to prime the tubing before attaching the light blue stopper tube.

CHAPTER 3

Review Questions

1. C
2. B
3. A
4. D
5. A
6. B
7. D
8. C
9. C
10. B

For Further Study

1. a. Not acceptable. The patient may become faint or dizzy during the procedure and collapse on the floor.
   b. Acceptable. The tourniquet would be applied too long if the equipment was not assembled first.
   c. Not acceptable. This will cause hemoconcentration of the sample.
   d. Acceptable. This provides maximum bacteriostatic cleansing at the actual puncture site.
   e. Not acceptable. This enlarges the puncture hole, possibly causing a hematoma.
2. a. A hematoma: Bending the patient's arm when applying pressure.
   b. Petechiae: Leaving the tourniquet on too tightly for too long.
   c. A patient to choke: Allowing the patient to have gum, a thermometer, or other item in his or her mouth while performing venipuncture.
   d. Blood to stop flowing when a tube is changed: The needle has moved either through the vein or out of the vein.
   e. Blood drops on a patient's slacks when the needle is removed: Failure to remove the last tube from the holder before removing the needle from the vein.
3. a. Determine the depth of the vein.
   b. Determine the size of the vein.
   c. Determine the direction of the vein.
4. a. Hemoconcentration might cause high molecular weight analytes to have erroneous results.

b. Hemolysis might occur, causing erroneously high potassium values.

Case Study 3-1

1. a. Improper patient identification.
   b. Tourniquet was not released while assembling the equipment and cleansing the site.
   c. Labeling the tube before blood collection.
   d. Blowing on the site to dry the alcohol.
2. a. The wrong patient may have had blood drawn or the tube mislabled that could cause treatment errors based on the laboratory results.
   b. Hemoconcentration might cause the high molecular weight analytes to have erroneous results because the tourniquet was on too long.
   c. Microbes could be introduced into the site because the blood collector contaminated the site by blowing on it.
3. The blood collector may be charged with malpractice if a patient received inappropriate treatment based on inaccurate results.

Case Study 3-2

1. The blood collector should ask on which side she had the mastectomy.
2. a. Lymphedema
   b. Infection
3. a. Increased blood level of lymphocytes.
   b. Contamination of sample with waste products contained in the lymph fluid.

CHAPTER 4

Review Questions

1. D
2. A
3. C
4. D
5. C
6. A
7. D
8. C
9. D
10. a. 3
    b. 4
    c. 1
    d. 2

For Further Study

1. Redirect the needle in only a forward or backward direction, try another light blue stopper tube, and if unsuccessful, request another blood collector to collect the sample.
2. The needle could have moved out of the vein. Slowly advance the needle into the vein if the needle is only partially in the lumen of the vein.
   Pull back on a needle that may have gone through the vein.
3. A hematoma is forming under the skin. Immediately release the tourniquet and remove the needle. Apply pressure to the site until bleeding has stopped. Re-collect the sample from the other arm with a 23-gauge needle using a winged blood collection set attached to a syringe.

Case Study 4-1

1. The needle may have touched a nerve.
2. The CLSI recommended needle angle is 15 to 30 degrees with the bevel up. The basilic vein should be only used as a last choice and after having checked both arms for an acceptable median cubital or cephalic vein. A needle angle of greater than 30 degrees should never be employed.
3. The sample might be hemolyzed because of the extensive probing, causing the laboratory to reject the sample.

Case Study 4-2

1. The sample contained small clots.
2. The blood collector was busy with the patient and did not mix the sample.
3. Yes. Use one hand to mix the sample as soon as the patient's head was lowered.

CHAPTER 5

Review Questions

1. C
2. D
3. B
4. C
5. D
6. C
7. C
8. B

9. D
10. C

For Further Study

1. Glucose levels are higher in capillary blood collected by dermal puncture than they are in venous blood.
2. Yes. Bilirubin is rapidly destroyed by light. The tube should have been protected from the light by covering the tube with aluminum foil.
3. The fasting blood sample is tested before administering the glucose to determine whether the patient can safely be given a large amount of glucose.
4. The patient should have been instructed to come to the laboratory early in the morning after a 12-hour fast.

Case Study 5-1

1. Yes. The concentration of microorganisms fluctuates and is highest before the patient's temperature spikes.
2. When the blood is collected using a winged blood collection set, the anaerobic bottle is inoculated second so that air does not enter the bottle.
3. Improper site cleansing when the first set was drawn.
4. False-negative cultures. Microorganisms present in the sample may be consumed in the microclots that can occur if the sample is not inverted.

Case Study 5-2

1. The color of the blood.
2. The brachial artery.
3. The blood collector should apply pressure for at least 5 minutes or until the bleeding has stopped.
4. A hematoma.

CHAPTER 6

Review Questions

1. C
2. B
3. B
4. D
5. B
6. C
7. A
8. A
9. B
10. A

For Further Study

1. Hemolysis.
2. No. The concentration of glucose is higher in blood obtained by dermal puncture.
3. Bilirubin is very sensitive to light and deteriorates quickly if not protected from the light.
4. a. Performing a dermal puncture on the back of the heel (calcaneous).
   b. Performing a dermal puncture on the sides or tips of the fingers.

Case Study 6-1

1. The alcohol should be allowed to dry and the first drop wiped away. Failure to let the alcohol dry on the puncture site produces hemolysis.
2. Scraping the skin to collect blood flowing down the finger will cause hemolysis.
3. Yes. A second puncture should be performed with a new lancet and new collection container. If blood from a second puncture is added to the first microcollection container, hemolysis and microclots might be present.

Case Study 6-2

1. Yes.
2. The lavender microcollection container should be collected first because platelets immediately begin adhering to the puncture site.
3. Excessive squeezing of the site or vigorous mixing of the sample.

CHAPTER 7

Review Questions

1. D
2. B
3. D
4. C
5. D
6. B
7. B
8. D
9. D
10. D

For Further Study

1. Normal and abnormal controls are performed to ensure that the testing system, reagents, and the person performing the test provide reliable results. QC must be acceptable before patient results are reported.
2. The QC testing is not within acceptable limits. A technical service representative must be contacted.
3. a. Unacceptable. Microscopic analysis of urine is classified as a PPMP and not a waived test.
   b. Acceptable.
   c. Unacceptable. The sample must dry on the slide for 3 to 5 minutes.
   d. Unacceptable. Cartridges and extraction solution must come from the same kit. Reagents from different manufacturers are not interchangeable.

Case Study 7-1

1. No.
2. Rerun the QC using a new abnormal high control.
3. The abnormal high control could be outdated or contaminated. The test strip could be outdated or contaminated. Test strips and analyzer code number don't match.

Case Study 7-2

1. Bacteria in the sample could have multiplied.
2. It should have been refrigerated when it cannot be tested within 2 hours.
3. Ask the patient for another sample.

CHAPTER 8

Review Questions

1. B
2. C
3. B
4. B
5. A
6. D
7. B
8. C
9. A
10. A

For Further Study

1. a. Pulling the plunger of the syringe too rapidly.
   b. Forcing blood from the syringe into an evacuated tube.
2. Syringes filled with sterile saline are used to prime a collection stopcock or clear a line prior to collecting blood or infusing a different substance into a line that has already been infusing a medication or treatment. Flush syringes clear a line following blood collection to avoid occlusion of the line by allowing blood to clot in the line.
3. There must be 20 mL of blood discarded before obtaining the coagulation sample.
4. The blood collector must have knowledge of the various CVD collecting devices, flush protocols, and sterile technique. IV lines provide a direct path for infectious organisms to enter the patient's bloodstream.

Case Study 8-1

1. Aspirate a 5-mL waste and discard.
2. Two 10-mL syringes and two 5-mL syringes.
3. A transfer device will be attached to the syringe.
4. Light green, lavender, and light blue, which is collected last using a new syringe.

Case Study 8-2

1. The line draw was contaminated with heparin.
2. Heparin and saline.
3. The flush protocol is to flush two or three times the amount of the line (18 to 19 mL).
4. 20 mL.

Laboratory Abbreviations Commonly Used

AABB	American Association of Blood Banks
Ab	Antibody
ABGs	Arterial blood gases
ABO	Blood group
ACD	Acid citrate dextrose
ACT	Activated clotting time
ACTH	Adrenocorticotropic hormone
ADA	American Diabetes Association
ADH	Antidiuretic hormone
Ag	Antigen
AIDS	Acquired immunodeficiency syndrome
ALP	Alkaline phosphatase
ALT	Alanine aminotransferase
ANA	Antinuclear antibody
APTT (PTT)	Activated partial thromboplastin time
ARD	Antimicrobial removal device
ASAP	As soon as possible
ASCP	American Society for Clinical Pathology
ASO	Antistreptolysin O
AST	Aspartate aminotransferase
BB	Blood bank
BNP	Brain natriuretic peptide
BP	Blood pressure
BSI	Body substance isolation
BT	Bleeding time
BUN	Blood urea nitrogen
C & S	Culture and sensitivity
Ca	Calcium
CAP	College of American Pathologists
CBC	Complete blood count
CBGs	Capillary blood gases
CDC	Centers for Disease Control and Prevention
CEA	Carcinoembryonic antigen
CK	Creatine kinase
CK-BB, MB, MM	Creatine kinase isoenzymes
Cl	Chloride
CLSI	Clinical and Laboratory Standards Institute
cm	Centimeter
CMS	Centers for Medicare & Medicaid Services
CNA	Certified Nursing Assistant
CO_2	Carbon dioxide
COC	Chain of custody
COLA	Commission on Laboratory Assessment
COPD	Chronic obstructive pulmonary disease
CPR	Cardiopulmonary resuscitation
CPT	Certified Phlebotomy Technician
CRP	C-reactive protein
ctO_2	Oxygen content
CVAD	Central venous access device
DAT	Direct antihuman globulin test
DIC	Disseminated intravascular coagulation
Diff	Differential
DM	Diabetes mellitus
DOB	Date of birth
Dx	Diagnosis
ED	Emergency department
EDTA	Ethylenediaminetetraacetic acid
EMLA	Eutectic mixture of local anesthetics
ESR	Erythrocyte sedimentation rate
ETS	Evacuated tube system
FANA	Fluorescent antinuclear antibody
FDA	Food and Drug Administration
FDP	Fibrin degradation product
FIo_2	Fraction of inspired oxygen

FSH	Follicle-stimulating hormone	OSHA	Occupational Safety and Health Administration
FTA-ABS	Fluorescent treponemal antibody—absorbed	P	Phosphorus
FUO	Fever of unknown origin	PAP	Prostatic acid phosphatase
g, gm	Gram	PBT	Phlebotomy Technician
GGT	Gamma-glutamyl transferase	P_{CO_2}	Partial pressure of carbon dioxide
GH	Growth hormone	PEP	Postexposure prophylaxis
GI	Gastrointestinal	PF3	Platelet factor 3
GTT	Glucose tolerance test	pH	Negative log of the hydrogen ion concentration (less than 7 is acid and above 7 is alkaline)
HAI	Healthcare–associated infection		
HBIg	Hepatitis B immune globulin		
HbsAg	Hepatitis B surface antigen	PICC	Peripherally inserted central catheter
HBV	Hepatitis B virus	PKU	Phenylketonuria
HCG	Human chorionic gonadotropin	Plt	Platelet
HCl	Hydrochloric acid	P_{O_2}	Partial pressure of oxygen
HCO_3	Bicarbonate	POC	Point of care
Hct	Hematocrit	POCT	Point-of-care testing
HCV	Hepatitis C virus	pp	Postprandial
HDL	High-density lipoprotein	PPE	Personal protective equipment
HDN	Hemolytic disease of the newborn	PPMP	Provider-performed microscopy procedures
Hgb	Hemoglobin		
HIPAA	Health Insurance Portability and Accountability Act of 1996	PPT	Plasma preparation tube
		PSA	Prostate-specific antigen
HIV	Human immunodeficiency virus	PST	Plasma separator tube
HLA	Human leukocyte antigen	PT	Prothrombin time
Ig	Immunoglobulin	PTH	Parathyroid hormone
IM	Intramuscular	QA	Quality assurance
IM	Infectious mononucleosis	QC	Quality control
INR	International normalized ratio	QM	Quality management
IRDS	Infant respiratory distress syndrome	QNS	Quantity nonsufficient
ISO	International Standardization Organization	RA	Rheumatoid arthritis
		RBC	Red blood cell
IV	Intravenous	RDW	Red blood cell distribution width
K	potassium	Retic	Reticulocyte
K_2EDTA	Dipotassium ethylenediaminetetraacetic acid	RF	Rheumatoid factor
		RFID	Radio frequency identification
K_3EDTA	Tripotassium ethylenediaminetetraacetic acid	Rh	The D (Rhesus) antigen on red blood cells
		RIA	Radioimmunoassay
kg	Kilogram	RPR	Rapid plasma reagin
LD	Lactate dehydrogenase	SDS	Safety Data Sheets
LDL	Low-density lipoprotein	SLE	Systemic lupus erythematosus
LH	Luteinizing hormone	SP	Standard precautions
Li	Lithium	SPS	Sodium polyanethol sulfonate
LIS	Laboratory information system	SST	Serum separator tube
Lytes	Electrolytes	stat	Immediately
MCH	Mean corpuscular hemoglobin	T & C	Type and crossmatch
MCHC	Mean corpuscular hemoglobin concentration	T_3	Triiodothyronine
		T_4	Thyroxine
MCV	Mean corpuscular volume	TAT	Turnaround time
mg	Milligram	TC/HDL	Total cholesterol/high-density lipoprotein
Mg	Magnesium	TDM	Therapeutic drug monitoring
MI	Myocardial infarction	TIBC	Total iron binding capacity
mL	Milliliter	TJC	The Joint Commission
MLS	Medical Laboratory Scientist	TP	Total protein
MLT	Medical Laboratory Technician	TPN	Total parenteral nutrition (IV feeding)
mm	Millimeter	TSH	Thyroid-stimulating hormone
mm Hg	Millimeters of mercury	TT	Thrombin time
MSH	Melanocyte-stimulating hormone	VDRL	Venereal Disease Research Laboratory
Na	Sodium	VLDL	Very low-density lipoprotein
O_2	Oxygen	WBC	White blood cell
O_2Sat	Oxygen saturation	WHO	World Health Organization
OGTT	Oral glucose tolerance test	ZDV	Zidovudine
OP	Outpatient		

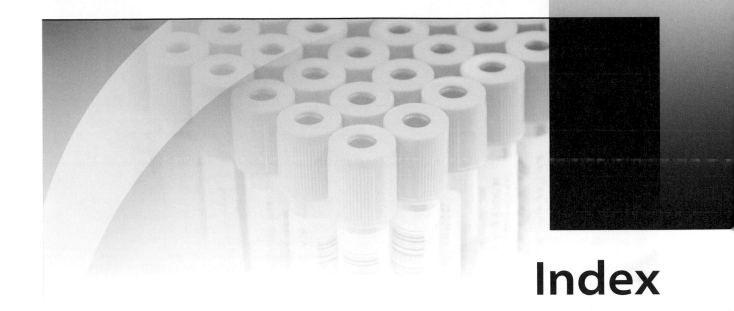

Index

Page numbers followed by "f" denote figures; "b" denote boxes; and "t" denote tables

BD Vacutainer Venous Blood Collection Tube Guide

Hemogard™ Closure	Conventional Stopper	Additive	Inv	Laboratory Use	Notes
Gold	Red/Gray	• Clot activator and gel for serum separation	5	For serum determinations in chemistry. Blood clotting time: 30 minutes.	
Light Green	Green/Gray	• Lithium heparin and gel for plasma separation	8	For plasma determinations in chemistry.	
Red	Red	• Silicone coated (glass) • Clot activator, silicone coated (plastic)	0 5	For serum determinations in chemistry. Blood clotting time, glass: 60 minutes. Blood clotting time, plastic: 30 minutes.	
Orange		• Thrombin-based clot activator with gel for serum separation	5 to 6	For stat serum determinations in chemistry. Blood clotting time: 5 minutes.	
Orange		• Thrombin-based clot activator	8	For stat serum determinations in chemistry. Blood clotting time: 5 minutes.	
Royal Blue		• Clot activator (plastic serum) • K_2EDTA (plastic)	5 8	For trace-element, toxicology, and nutritional-chemistry determinations.	
Green	Green	• Sodium heparin • Lithium heparin	8 8	For plasma determinations in chemistry.	
Gray	Gray	• Potassium oxalate/sodium fluoride • Sodium fluoride/Na_2 EDTA • Sodium fluoride (serum tube)	8 8 8	For glucose determinations.	
Tan		• K_2EDTA (plastic)	8	For lead determinations.	
Lavender	Lavender	• Liquid K_3EDTA (glass) • Spray-coated K_2EDTA (plastic)	8 8	For whole blood hematology determinations.	
	Yellow	• Sodium polyanethol sulfonate (SPS) • Acid citrate dextrose additives (ACD): **Solution A** 22.0 g/L trisodium citrate, 8.0 g/L citric acid, 24.5 g/L dextrose **Solution B** 13.2 g/L trisodium citrate, 4.8 g/L citric acid, 14.7 g/L dextrose	8 8 8	SPS for blood culture specimens in microbiology. ACD for blood bank studies, HLA phenotyping, and DNA and paternity testing.	
White		• K_2EDTA and gel for plasma separation	8	For use in molecular diagnostic test methods.	
Pink	Pink	• Spray-coated K_2EDTA (plastic)	8	For whole blood immunohematology testing. Special cross-match label.	
Light Blue Clear	Light Blue Light Blue	• Buffered sodium citrate 0.105 M (3.2%) glass 0.109 M (3.2%) plastic • Citrate, theophylline, adenosine, dipyridamole (CTAD)	3–4 3–4	For coagulation determinations.	
Clear	Red/Light Gray	• None (plastic)	0	For use as a discard tube or secondary specimen tube.	

Courtesy and © Becton, Dickinson and Company. Adapted with permission.   *Inversions at blood collection